Migraines FOR DUMMIES®

POCKET EDITION

by Diane Stafford and Jennifer Shoquist, MD

Look for Pocket Editions on these other topics:

Allergies For Dummies, Pocket Edition
Anxiety & Depression For Dummies, Pocket Edition
Asthma For Dummies, Pocket Edition
Diabetes For Dummies, Pocket Edition
Dieting For Dummies, Pocket Edition
Heart Disease For Dummies, Pocket Edition
High Blood Pressure For Dummies, Pocket Edition
Menopause For Dummies, Pocket Edition

WILEY

Wiley Publishing, Inc.

Migraines For Dummies,® Pocket Edition

Published by
Wiley Publishing, Inc.
111 River St.
Hoboken, NJ 07030-5774
www.wiley.com

For general information on our other products and services, please contact our Customer Care Department within the U.S. at 800-762-2974, outside the U.S. at 317-572-3993, or fax 317-572-4002.

For technical support, please visit www.wiley.com/techsupport.

Wiley also publishes its books in a variety of electronic formats. Some content that appears in print may not be available in electronic books.

Library of Congress Control Number: 2005936647

ISBN-13: 978-0-471-79234-5

ISBN-10: 0-471-79234-9

Manufactured in the United States of America

10 9 8 7 6 5 4 3 2 1

1O/RS/QR/QW/IN

Publisher's Acknowledgements

Project Editor: Elizabeth Kuball
Composition Services: Indianapolis Composition Services Department
Cover Photo: © Bruce Ayres/Getty Images

Table of Contents

• •

Introduction

● ●

About 28 million Americans have migraine headaches. And, if you're one of them, you know all too well that it's hard to predict what a day will hold. Any morning, afternoon, or evening, you may find yourself in the throes of mind-boggling pain, not to mention nausea, vomiting, and sensitivity to loud noises.

Migraines have been driving people nuts forever. Ancient "caregivers" bored holes in people's heads to try to relieve headache pain. Egyptians tied an herb-stuffed clay crocodile to an aching head.

Yet despite a history of being guinea pigs, migraine sufferers remain optimistic. Migraines hurt and can be very disabling, so bring on the remedies!

Knowledge is a powerful weapon in any fight and, in this book, we aim to arm you with the tools you need to whip your migraines into submission.

About This Book

Migraines For Dummies provides headache information that helps you understand what you're up against — and a list of remedies effective enough to merit high-roller status in any migraine circle in the world.

Migraines For Dummies offers hope, with a focused, fleshed-out program that works in the real world. Headache medications have their place in the picture, but you absolutely can do more.

The quest for answers — and the pilgrimage to a better health place — is at the core of this book. The migraine mob needs health advocates. And we, the authors of *Migraines For Dummies,* fill that role, offering valuable tips on ways to eliminate the fisticuffs going on inside your head in the wacky world of managed health care.

This book contains our opinions and ideas. We intend to provide helpful information on migraines, but we don't offer professional medical, health, or any other kind of personal services via the book.

Remember: This is a supplement, not a replacement, for medical advice from your personal healthcare provider. In no way does reading this book replace the need for an evaluation by a physician.

If you want or need personal advice or guidance, please consult a medical, health, or other competent professional — especially if you have a condition that may require medical diagnosis or attention — before adopting any of the suggestions in the book or drawing inferences from the information given.

Foolish Assumptions

Because you picked up this book, we assume a few things about you:

- ✔ You think that you have migraines, know that you have migraines, or live with, and love, someone with migraines.

 You're familiar with the debilitating factor, and you're looking for ideas that will be inspiring, instructive, and winning.

- ✔ You may have yet to find a remedy that gets rid of your head pain.

✔ You find the entire migraine problem and its related issues (work, family, public skepticism) somewhat daunting.

✔ You're baffled, unsure of what to do and when to do it.

✔ Our biggest assumption is that you're itching to discover ways to get rid of migraine pain, and we think that you can definitely find what you need in this book. We present clear and comprehensive information about all aspects of migraines, along with tips, encouragement, and reassurance.

Icons Used in This Book

For Dummies books use snazzy pictures in the margins to draw your attention to specific bits of text. In this book, the pictures we use are

 When you see this icon, you'll find stories about how other migraineurs have coped.

 Tack this tidbit on your bulletin board!

 Paragraphs flagged by this icon caution you about practices and procedures you should talk to a doctor about and tell you when you should head for the emergency room.

 The dry medical info that you may or may not be interested in is highlighted with this icon. You can skip it if you like.

 This icon says: "Here's a valuable morsel you may want to read several times."

 This icon alerts you to danger signs and practices to avoid.

Where to Go from Here

With the intros tucked away, we usher you into the meat of the book. If your headaches haven't been diagnosed, start with Chapters 1 and 3, which acquaint you with the different types of headaches. Head to Chapter 2 to get a feel for when your migraines hit and what may be triggering them. Check out Chapters 4, 5, and 6 to find out how to deal with your migraines medically, practically, and socially. And head to Chapter 7 for some "treatments" to avoid.

If you want even more information on migraines, from finding the right doctor for you to dealing with less-than-supportive folk, check out the full-size version of *Migraines For Dummies* — simply head to your local bookseller or go to www.dummies.com!

Chapter 1

Knowing What You're Dealing With: An Overview

● ●

In This Chapter

▶ Understanding migraines and other headaches

▶ Finding causes and triggers

▶ Seeing a specialist

▶ Taking on family and work issues

▶ Looking at various treatment options

● ●

About 28 million Americans have migraine headaches. According to the National Headache Foundation's report on the American Migraine Study II, about 53 percent of migraine sufferers have headache pain that causes severe impairment or forces them to retreat to bed. And, the Excedrin Headache Resource Center reports that more than 80 percent of *migraineurs* (people who get migraine headaches) have at least some headache-related disability; 50 percent or more, mild or moderate disability (inability to work or do usual activities); and 30 percent, severe disability. By age 15, about 75 percent of children have had a significant headache, and 28 percent of girls 15 to 19 appear to have migraines, according to *Headache and Migraine in Childhood and Adolescence,* edited by Vincenzo Guidetti, George Russell, Matti Sillanpaa, and Paul Winner.

Unfortunately, migraines cause children to miss school and adults to miss work. In fact, some employers grow so leery of migraine-ridden employees that they look askance at this kind of problem. To them, it translates to diminished attendance and low productivity. And, according to a study published in *Archives of Internal Medicine* (April 1999), employers have reason for their interpretation: The study cited migraine costs of $13 billion a year for American employers due to employees' missed work and lower productivity.

Getting a Take on What Migraines Are and What They Aren't

Migraines are intense, recurring headaches, but they aren't always debilitating, and they usually are manageable — if you take the time to sort out what kinds of things trigger your migraines, and what sorts of medications and lifestyle changes can make a big difference.

What migraines are

A common myth states that any bad headache, by virtue of being excruciating, must be a migraine. The truth, however, is that some migraines are mild to moderate (although many are severe, indeed). Some other types of headaches — tension-type headaches, for example — can be extremely painful, too, as can headaches caused by more serious problems such as a _hemorrhage_ (bleeding) in the brain.

The symptoms for migraines may take on many different traits in different people. The uniqueness of the symptoms, in fact, is one reason that some migraineurs end up living for years without appropriate and effective medication at hand — they don't realize that their headaches are, in fact, migraines.

For example, you may assume, based on what you've heard or what "everyone says," that the headaches you get simply can't be migraines because you don't experience the symptoms that those old wives of old-wives'-tale fame say make a headache a migraine. The truth, however, is that migraines have a wide variety of symptoms, and not every migraine sufferer has the classic symptoms.

Symptoms of migraine headaches include, but are not limited to the following:

- ✔ You feel a throbbing or hammering pain on one or both sides of your head.

- ✔ The pain ranges from moderate to severe to almost intolerable.

- ✔ You may experience an _aura_ (typically, a visual disturbance that lasts from a few minutes to less than an hour, or numbness and tingling of the mouth area and arms), although it's more common that migraine sufferers don't experience auras. Auras usually take place an hour or less before the headache.

- ✔ When you have a headache, you may feel lethargic and sad.

- ✔ Along with the headache, you may experience nausea, vomiting, malaise, an extreme sensitivity to light, smells, and/or sounds, and periods of no appetite.

Generally speaking, the following are some key features that characterize migraine sufferers:

- ✔ You come from a family that has other migraine-prone family members — your parents, grandparents, or siblings.

- ✔ Your headaches can last from several hours to two or three days.

- ✔ Sleep usually helps you feel better.

Your headache frequency can be several times a week, once a month, or even less often than that. And migraines can make their presence felt before and after the actual headache. A day or two before your headache, you may experience symptoms such as yawning, frequent urination, drowsiness, irritability, and/or euphoria. After a headache, you may experience a *pain hangover* — you're tired, you don't feel hungry, and your thinking process seems slower.

A migraine is essentially a headache and more. Because your central nervous system's normal state of functioning is disrupted during a migraine, all your body systems are affected. As a result, you may be bothered by sounds, smells, and lights, or your scalp may feel tender, or your feet and hands may be cold.

It's widely agreed that the symptoms of migraines can be different for each individual, so don't assume that your headaches aren't migraines just because you lack auras or other classic symptoms. For example, you may describe your pain as "splitting," while the classic symptom is more of a "throbbing" headache. You may happen to have generalized head pain instead of the classic one-sided misery. Or, you may have never experienced visual disturbances, nausea, or vomiting. Most migraineurs do experience light

sensitivity, but maybe you never have. So tell
your doctor about your symptoms, and let her
be the one to identify the kind of headaches
you're suffering from and determine what can
be done to wipe out the pain.

In many people, migraines occur because they have a
genetic tendency to get headaches — a body-system
glitch leads to neurochemical changes that spiral,
resulting in chemical shenanigans that affect blood
vessels, altering blood flow to your brain and causing
your head to ache (see Chapter 2).

Keeping the faith

Sometimes it takes a while to realize that the headaches
you're experiencing are migraines. One guy looked for help
for his horrible migraines for years. He had riveting pain that
was "like a jackhammer," and it took two or three days for
him to come out of the pain and fog. He went to bed in a
darkened room, and his daughter brought him fast food and
drinks until he felt better.

Finally, after living with migraines for ten years, he went to a
headache specialist. The headache specialist got him involved
in working up a regimen for pain relief. The prescription medication (a triptan) worked far better than anything he had taken
in the past. (For info about medications, see Chapter 5.) He
used relaxation techniques and began doing weight training.
Today, although he still has them occasionally, his headaches
are less debilitating, and he finally feels like he "has a life."

His biggest regret is that he waited so long to look for genuine
solutions. He just tried to grit his teeth and bear the pain.
"I thought having migraines was unmanly, so I suffered for
years just because of the stigma. I didn't want my doctor to
think I was a total wimp."

What migraines aren't

The other main types of headaches have symptoms that are different from those of migraines — but sometimes symptoms overlap, making diagnosis difficult. (See Chapter 3 for information on headaches often confused with migraines.)

Some signs that your headache *isn't* a migraine:

> ✔ Your head pain can best be described as a dull ache.
>
> ✔ Your shoulder and neck muscles feel knotted up.
>
> ✔ You have headaches only after sex or physical exertion.
>
> ✔ Your headaches are getting steadily worse.

Tripping through the Types of Headaches

Consider the following indicators of these common headache types.

Migraines

The key symptoms that most healthcare providers look for are a throbbing head pain that's typically one-sided, intensity that's moderate to severe, and a lengthy duration (migraines can range from a few hours up to several days). Activity may make you feel even worse. You may have accompanying nausea and vomiting, and/or sensitivity to light and sound. If you suffer from migraines, you usually have headaches on a regular basis.

Comparing migraines with auras to ones without

A relatively small percentage (about 20 percent) of migraine sufferers have the signals or symptoms called *auras* (visual disturbances, speech problems, distortions of smells and sounds, numb hands, feet, and lips). Some migraineurs have auras occasionally, while others have never had a single aura during their histories of headaches.

Most migraineurs don't experience auras. So if your headaches don't come with auras, you aren't automatically placed in a different headache category (contrary to popular belief).

Tension-type headaches

With this type of headache, you have a dull ache characterized by mild to moderate pain. The aching is on both sides of your head, and it comes on slowly.

If you feel pain around your neck and the back of your head, or in the forehead and temple region — and if the pain feels more like tightness than it does a throbbing or pounding — then you probably have a tension-type headache. You won't have nausea or auras with this kind of headache. Tension-type headaches can occur very frequently (even daily) and are sometimes very painful.

Cluster headaches

This headache is characterized by sudden and severe piercing pain on one side of the head. These headaches come in clusters — appearing during several consecutive days, weeks, or months, and then disappearing,

only to come back months or years later. Cluster headaches can come and go five or six times during a day.
They're usually short-lived, lasting from 30 minutes to
two or three hours each time.

With a cluster headache, you may have a droopy-
looking eyelid or sweating on the side that hurts,
and you may find that moving around makes you feel
better. Typically, cluster headaches aren't accompa-
nied by nausea or vomiting. Pain comes from behind
one eye. The eye may tear up or become red, and the
nostril on this same side may run or feel congested.

Looking at Some of the Reasons Why

If migraines run in your family, you may well have inherited a migraine tendency, which means that your gene
pool set you up with a super-sensitive nervous system.
Along with the hair you love and the nose you loathe,
your predilection for migraines is part of your genetic
material, and you can't run away from it. (Chapter 2
has more on the genetics/migraine connection.)

A migraine tendency is a dominant trait, so you
probably inherited the penchant for having
these headaches from your parent who suffers
from migraines.

You may have noticed that certain foods, activities,
sounds, or smells seem to trigger migraines. The
problem is, this expected result may not occur every
single time you eat Chinese food or take an aerobics
class. It usually takes a village of triggers to raise a
migraine: You never know if or when they're going to
team up.

Getting an Under-the-Hood Inspection and Tune-Up

Diagnosing and treating migraines may require an investment of time, money, patience, trial-and-error, journaling (to discover triggers), and a strong working relationship with a doctor who does headache diagnosis.

Getting to the bottom of headaches can be complicated, so don't try to go it alone. If you do, chances are you'll flounder around for years without coming to any firm conclusions or finding painkillers that serve your needs.

After you've been diagnosed with migraines, you can take your place as the Sultan of Scathing Headaches, starting to put remedies to work and implementing lifestyle changes. Find a positive tilt for the family and work issues associated with your headaches, and discover the best things to do when pain hits. You should also try to find ways to keep a migraine from forming.

Aspects of migraine management include:

- ✔ Finding the right doctor and creating a treatment strategy
- ✔ Working to eliminate migraine triggers
- ✔ Handling family and work issues
- ✔ Getting a heads-up on special issues, such as migraines associated with seniors, women, kids, stress, and sex
- ✔ Familiarizing yourself with red-flag headache signs that should send you scurrying to the emergency room

Most of the time, migraines are quite manageable. Just figure out your headache triggers and rearrange certain aspects of your lifestyle, and you'll be on the road to sending your headaches to the B-team bench, where they'll languish and rarely take a starring role again.

Call on your top-flight patience when you start trying migraine treatments. Although you may get lucky and find that the first migraine drug your doctor recommends works perfectly for you, it's more common to have to go through a trial-and-error period of testing medications.

Migraines are quirky. If they weren't, doctors would be able to recommend the one super-sized honcho power-pill, and there would be no need for a book called *Migraines For Dummies*. But the truth is, migraine headaches come in as many varieties as there are materials in a fabric store. This variety makes them difficult — but certainly not impossible — to treat.

Handling Family and Work Issues

Getting a handle on family and work issues associated with migraines has several advantages. For one thing, you miss less work or school after you zero in on successful ways to manage your headaches. At the same time, though, the chronic nature of migraines means that you need to be prepared to deal with a headache that strikes when you're outside the home. You must have an arsenal of techniques ready to go.

Also, the people skills involved in migraine management are extremely important because people who don't have migraines usually have trouble understanding them or relating to the sometimes-debilitating nature of headaches.

Dealing with being misunderstood

Try really hard to understand all those folks who don't have migraines. You may wonder, "Why? What do you mean?" You may also feel indignant, "Hey, wait a minute — shouldn't *I* be the one expecting understanding?"

Well, the main reason you need to walk in others' shoes is because they definitely won't understand you or your headache predicament. Migraines are a strange illness to an outsider, and you really can't expect someone who hasn't had one to understand much about them.

Most people who are migraine-free view migraine headaches in one or more of the following ways:

- **With skepticism:** They think that you're a hypochondriac.
- **With empathy:** They're sorry that you have to suffer.
- **With disinterest:** They don't want to hear about your migraines.
- **With anger:** They're mad when you have to cancel or call in sick, and your migraines inconvenience them.
- **With confusion:** Children, for example, have trouble understanding why a parent sometimes gets sick and can't do things for them, or why family activities have to be cancelled.

Taking these facts into consideration will help you deal with people around you in a happier, more consistent way. In return, you'll get better treatment because those close to you will know what to expect.

If head pain were your one-and-only problem, you'd
be looking at a very different kind of malady. But the
truth is, everyone associated with a migraineur is
affected in some way (or to some degree) by the long-
term nature of the affliction. It's up to you to set the
tone for deft handling of your migraine's "extended
family" of issues with all the people you deal with —
family, friends, co-workers.

Basically, you either establish yourself as a
capable, reliable individual who just happens to
have headaches from time to time, or as a dis-
abled person who wants everyone around her
to jump when she needs help and show massive
amounts of sympathy when she's down and out.

Exploring Options Galore

Without a doubt, the treatment/management situation
today is very promising for migraine sufferers. You
have much to celebrate. You have more options than
your mother or grandmother had when she was nurs-
ing a headache. These options can help make your life
easier and much more enjoyable.

The following advantages represent the final word on
today's overall migraine picture:

✔ **Doctors know much more about migraines
   than they did 20 years ago.** The introduction of
   triptan migraine drugs, specifically, improved
   the migraine-treatment picture dramatically
   (see Chapter 5 for more on prescription drugs).

✔ **Healthcare providers take migraines seriously.**
   They can guide migraine sufferers in eliminating
   lifestyle factors that can aggravate a highly sensitive nervous system. The upshot: The migraineur
   is able to become less dependent on medication.

- ✔ **The drug options for treating migraines are head and shoulders above the ones that were available a few decades ago.** Today's medications are way more effective because some of them are migraine-specific.

- ✔ **Alternative therapies abound.** And some of these may serve as excellent complements to your primary migraine-management plan.

- ✔ **Generally speaking, most people have more-accepting attitudes about the severity of migraines, even though headaches remain shrouded in some degree of mystery.**

- ✔ **Migraine sufferers have found a voice.** Most realize that they do, indeed, have a right to speak up and seek help.

Suffering in silence with a migraine has gone the way of pecking on a typewriter. Migraine treatment is now so smart and savvy that it represents multitasking at its best. Bill Gates would be proud. And you can be headache-free.

Chapter 2

Knowing Your Foes

. . . .

In This Chapter

▶ Cranking up your journaling skills

▶ Getting a handle on hereditary migraines

▶ Evaluating the environment for triggers

▶ Avoiding dietary triggers

▶ Knowing which exercises can lead to migraines

▶ Catching the odds-and-ends triggers

▶ Defeating triggers with lifestyle changes

. . . .

*W*hen head monsters are pounding nails into your neurons, you're ready to try anything. Before you grab a random remedy, however, try developing a headache-busting agenda where you check out the usual suspects. Start by creating a journal in which you keep up with the foods you eat and your lifestyle habits — all the time looking for problem areas that seem to contribute to headache evolution.

Doing a little detective work can help you zero in on your personal troublemakers. Certain aspects of your meals and your environment may be headache-causing "toxins," so the sooner you pinpoint these triggers, the quicker you can get a handle on the fate of your pain.

Keeping a Journal to Discover Reasons and Triggers

Who knew? You probably never figured that some day you'd be sitting in your living room with a spiral notebook or a handheld computer, making notes about the things you do, eat, smell, and hear on a quest to discover the weasels behind your migraines. If you prefer a ready-to-go itemizer: Copy the journal in Figure 2-1.

Whatever method you use to journal, the important step is to launch an intensive search for the Trigger Terrors that get together and conspire against you. These triggers are the ones that begin the trek down the road that leads to the mega-pain of a migraine headache.

When starting a journal, follow these basic steps:

1. **Carry your journal at all times.**

2. **Record what you eat, where you go, what the environment's like, and so on.**

   Check out Figure 2-1 for all the specifics of what you should jot down in your headache journal.

3. **Write down the specifics of any migraine —
   when it started, what it felt like, and so on —
   and the pattern of the pain you experience.**

   A pain pattern could be a migraine that occurs every four to five days and lasts about three hours each time, for example.

4. **Note the remedies you try and how effective they are.**

Journaling may strike you as time-consuming and, well, maybe a little bit *boring* . . . but hey, if it can put you back in the Game of Life, feeling good and rambunctious (with a head free of pain), it has to be well worth the minutes you devote to jotting down your pain patterns and possible triggers.

Headache Journal			
Onset and Duration	**Headache Traits**	**Possible Triggers**	**Remedies and Their Effectiveness**
Date of headache: Time since last headache: number of hours, days or weeks: Where were you when you got the headache: Signs that a headache was coming: visual disturbances, yawning, drowsiness, and so on. List all: Duration of headache: number of hours or days:	**Associated symptoms:** nausea, vomiting, light or sound sensitivity, and so on. List all: **Pain rating** on a scale of 1 (very little pain) to 10 (incapacitating pain): **Location of pain:** on side of the head, both sides, generalized, behind the eye, and so on. List all: **Type of pain:** throbbing, dull ache, sharp, band-like. List all: Does movement aggravate your headache? Is the pain: off and on or consistent?	**Emotions:** List anything especially exciting or anxiety-producing: **Hormones:** Indicate whether your headache was before, during, or after your period, and whether you're menopausal: **Food and drink:** List what you ate and drank. Include caffeine consumption and whether you consumed your usual amount at the usual time: **Alcohol/drug consumption:** List any alcohol or drugs you ingested: **Physical activity:** List what type of exercise you engaged in, including whether you had sex: **Environment:** Were you exposed to excessive sunlight or bright light: a change in the weather, a change in altitude, dust, smoke, and so on. List all:	**Remedies Tried** **Over-the-counter medication:** Advil, Excedrin, aspirin, and so on. List type and dosage: **Prescription medication:** List name and dosage: **Complementary remedies:** List method and how long you used it: How far into the headache did you try the treatment? **Effectiveness** **Medication:** Indicate, in hours, how long it took the medication to be effective, as well as whether it dulled the pain but didn't eliminate it, or didn't help at all: **Complementary remedy:** Indicate what effect the remedy had on your head pain and on your ability to cope with your migraine:

Figure 2-1: Sharing your headache journal can help your doctor treat your migraines.

A *trigger* is anything, whether internal or external, that sets a migraine attack in motion. Typically, you make a judgment call when identifying a trigger (is it a trigger or not?); after all, suspected triggers don't wear banners that say, "Hey, we're here to mess with you!" Plus, a specific trigger may not cause a headache every single time — instead, a specific combination of factors may be the catalyst.

At the end of each day, make a notation next to any item in your journal that seems to contribute to the development of a headache within 30 minutes to an hour. Track four or five separate headache days.

Things that seem to be triggers may actually only be coincidences; recording a number of headaches helps narrow things.

Understanding Inherited Migraines

You have beautiful turquoise eyes from your father, straight teeth from your grandmother, and an incredible singing voice from your grandfather — and, well, migraine headaches from your mother. (Of course, she feels really bad about it. But still, that little tag-you're-it came floating down in the gene pool when you were trolling for a set of traits, and now it's pretty much a done deal.) How can you inherit migraines? Well, nothing's truly set in stone on the migraine story, but many experts believe that a specific gene determines a person's proclivity for migraines.

A genetic predisposition for migraines in certain people appears to be a given. In fact, most migraineurs have a strong family history of agonizing head pain.

 Underscoring the theory of inheriting migraines is researchers' discovery of an area on chromosome 19 that relates to a certain kind of migraine. This finding points to a specific inherited pattern in families who have *hemiplegic migraine*. This headache types causes temporary paralysis on one side of the body. The paralysis, which occurs in your face, arm, or leg, can last from one hour to days, but it usually lasts for about 24 hours.

 You can't distinguish temporary weakness or paralysis from a stroke, so you need to be evaluated by a doctor who can consider all causes of acute onset weakness.

 You can inherit familial hemiplegic migraine if your family tree has at least two people who have migraines with aura that feature this one-sided weakness. So you may inherit the *tendency* to have migraines, but it takes your own personal trigger (or two or three) to set off a headache. Researchers regard the migraine tendency as a dominant trait. If one of your parents has migraines, you may inherit the proclivity. You're more likely to inherit it from your mother than your father.

A less common theory is that everyone in the world has the potential for migraines, but some people have a low threshold to triggers, whereas others have a high threshold. If you're a low-threshold type, your migraines trigger more easily than those of the high-threshold type.

Checking Your Environment for Allergens

Headache sufferers can be supersensitive to the content of their environments, so evaluating your own home and workplace for possible headache triggers is a good idea.

The following list provides some general tips for improving your environment:

- ✔ **Clean your indoor air by placing a negative-ion generator in your bedroom.**

- ✔ **Change air-conditioner filters frequently.**

- ✔ **Set houseplants around your rooms to filter indoor pollution.** Plants that horticulturists recommend for filtering air include aloe vera, ficus, philodendron, spider plants, and areca palms.

- ✔ **Have your tap water tested for impurities and carcinogens.**

- ✔ **Install a home water-purification unit or have bottled water delivered to your home.**

- ✔ **Look into the indoor air quality of places you frequent, such as your workplace.**

- ✔ **Hire an inspector to check your home for mold, pollens, bacteria, asbestos, radon, elevated levels of carbon monoxide, leaky gas furnaces, and noxious fumes.**

Finding Dietary Villains

Diet is a category that can make a major difference in the frequency and severity of your headaches. Most people who suffer from migraines have one or more triggers in the food-and-beverage genre. You just have to figure out which ones are yours.

Recording everything you eat and drink enables you to key in on the food/drink ogres that give you fits, so be sure that you don't leave out anything.

Foods and other things you ingest that may cause migraines include

- ✔ **Beverages, including alcohol, coffee, tea, and so on**
- ✔ **Foods you eat on the road (in the car, at movies, at friends' and relatives' homes):** When recording food triggers, most people don't include road foods, because they think that they have no control over what they eat away from home.
- ✔ **Meals and snacks**
- ✔ **Medications (prescription and over-the-counter), including hormone replacement therapy and birth control pills**
- ✔ **Vitamins**

Poor eating habits, such as failing to drink enough fluids (which can cause dehydration) and skipping meals, can also cause problems.

Leaving behind the dark, sweet stuff (reality therapy for chocoholics)

Here's the latest theory from the chocolate folks: After experts told us for decades that the dark, delicious stuff called chocolate was a migraine trigger, it has been determined that it's not true, after all.

As Emily Litella used to say on *Saturday Night Live:*
"Never mind!" Unfortunately, we can line up a
number of migraineurs who beg to disagree. For
them, chocolate does, indeed, seem to trigger
headaches.

You have to make your own call. Go ahead and dip into
that box of chocolates if you just can't resist — but go
into it with your eyes wide open. Truth be told, sometimes a food is so delicious that the taste-temptation
payoff is almost worth the headache. Almost. But not
quite.

As a general rule, if you're thrashing about for
answers to your migraines, eliminating chocolate for a while may be smart. If you find out
that chocolate is not a trigger, you can always
return to chocoholic heaven.

Checking for MSG on menus and labels

Here at the outset of migraine-busting, you need to
know that one of the most common food triggers for
migraine-prone folks is *monosodium glutamate* (MSG),
a flavor enhancer often added to Chinese foods and
also found in seasoning salt and other flavor enhancers.
Years ago, cooks commonly added MSG to veggies
to jazz them up (the stuff perks up the taste of food).
But soon those little shakers of MSG became less in
demand, as more and more people began to link
migraines to MSG. The bad rap was well deserved,
and, like a nickname, it stuck.

If you find that MSG does trigger your migraine headaches, become a good label reader. Develop a habit of checking for it in foods you buy, and be vigilant for other camouflaged words that let MSG sneak into your foods.

Some common aliases for MSG include

✔ sodium glutamate

✔ hydrolyzed protein

✔ calcium caseinate

✔ sodium caseinate

Some of the many places MSG may hide include the following:

✔ Asian foods in supermarkets

✔ Candy and gum

✔ Canned soups

✔ Chinese food in restaurants

✔ Dry-roasted nuts

✔ Flavorings such as soy sauce, broth, and bouillon

✔ Frozen dinners

✔ Iced tea mixes

✔ Meats packaged with sauces (sometimes)

✔ Packaged gravy

✔ Processed meats

✔ Some sports drinks and diet drinks

✔ Spices/seasonings

Zeroing In on Exercises That Make Your Head Hurt

You take a step aerobics class and end up paying for it with a migraine. You notice a trend: Every time you exercise vigorously, your head hurts afterward. Yes, exercise can trigger migraines in some folks, but don't give up on being a fitness enthusiast just because you've had some bad experiences. In fact, exercise can actually be used to help fend off headaches. You simply have to figure out which forms of exercise work for you and which forms trigger headaches.

Regular exercise three times a week for 30 to 45 minutes may actually ward off painful headache episodes. Movement increases your brain's production of *endorphins* — those well-known (and much talked about) chemical schmoozers that are both mood elevators and pain reducers.

If you suspect that exercise is a migraine trigger for you, list in your journal the length of time it takes you to warm up, the type of exercise you use, the duration of your workout, and how soon after the workout you develop a headache.

 Just keep in mind that the key element of a migraine sufferer's workout should be a slow, stretch-and-move warm-up prior to cutting loose.

Abandoning oh-that's-intense exercises

So, you love *Spinning* (an exercise where you pedal a stationary bike from low to high speeds to simulate uphill and downhill riding), or you can't get enough of the high-energy bench class at your health club, but you always walk away with a headache. *Hello!* These exercises are triggers for you!

The key word here is *acceptance.* You simply can't get your heart set on defining yourself as a super Spinner, an ace aerobics performer, or a champion triathlete if doing these workouts gives you grief (in other words, headaches) on a consistent basis.

Bypassing known terrors for kinder forms of exercise

The good news is that there are many kinds of exercises you *can* do. Use them as replacements for the tough-to-handle workouts that lead to headaches.

Try participating in a water exercise class or a low-impact aerobics class. Both are widely available at YMCAs, YWCAs, and health clubs.

Start a program of walking, swimming, yoga, Pilates, dance, or cycling. Sometimes you can make the pain go away by doing some slow-motion exercising when you feel the first twinges of a headache.

 Hydration is extra-important for exercisers who have a tendency to get migraines. Have your water bottle handy, and keep track of how much water you drink so you can make sure that you're getting enough. (Most days, you should drink about eight to ten 8-ounce glasses of water. Increase that amount by one glass per hour of vigorous, sweat-inducing exercise.) Sure, all that super-imbibing will have you trotting to the bathroom more often, but it's a small price to pay for staying headache-free.

Keying In on Other Migraine Triggers

So many triggers, so little time. But somehow your body is willing to work overtime in an effort to scrounge up gnarly reactions to many of the ordinary elements of everyday living.

So even if you're perfectly immune to most food and exercise triggers, don't start feeling too smug. A migraine thug may be waiting right around the corner, and you'll be in for big trouble when that trigger-happy thing stomps across your brain, toting a cartful of ammo.

If it's not one thing, it's another

Remember when Gilda Radner played the woe-ridden, jaw-chewing Roseanne Roseannadanna character, whose motto was "It's always something!" on *Saturday Night Live?*

You have to figure that she (or one of the show's comedy writers) had migraines — because, when it comes to migraines, it's always something. And, if it's not one thing, it's another.

A college freshman told us that she didn't understand why Chinese food would give her a headache one time she ate it, not have an effect on her the next time she ate it, and then have an effect on her again the third time. The matter got really confusing one night when she ate chocolate, which she nibbled frequently, and then got a horrible migraine. Until she ate that particular dessert (chocolate mousse), chocolate had never been a problem for her! Did the chocolate have a bad reaction with her birth control pills or the acetaminophen she had been taking all day?

Then she read an article about how triggers can team up to cause migraines. Although one thing alone (chocolate, for example) may not be enough to spur a headache, several things together may do the job. Until that point, she had worried that some things could just turn into demons overnight, leaving behind a killer headache for her to exorcise. Basically, what she called a "chocolate migraine" was really the result of a bunch of triggers forming a powerful posse and giving her head a wallop she'd never forget.

This young woman talked to her gynecologist, who had firsthand experience with migraine headaches. The doctor told her that triggers are sometimes so unpredictable that it seems as if a perfectly friendly thing (tea or peanut butter, for example) will suddenly sprout a devil's tail — and you end up with a really splitting headache that sends you to bed to sleep it off. The doctor also explained how sometimes certain things will bother you (and start a headache), and other times, they won't. "They have to get together with some buddies — other triggers — to cause a migraine, but all too often, that happens."

The doctor told her to track her food and lifestyle triggers in a headache journal. A few weeks later, she took her journal back to the doctor and got a prescription for a migraine medication that really helped her. In two hours, it knocked out a migraine! So she discovered that trigger-tracking was well worth the effort and time.

Sometimes even old friends seem to turn on you. Nontriggers convert to triggers — or at least, that's what you think is happening. Things that you've always tolerated well — medications, foods, exercise — get rebellious and go toxic one day for no apparent reason. So you're shocked when you develop a headache as an almost immediate response to something that you've lived in harmony with for years. Unfair and nonsensical! Yes, you're right on both counts — but it happens nonetheless.

The truth is, this is what probably happens in such cases: You have an onslaught of triggers acting together to cause a migraine — so it just *seems like* something benign and nontrigger-like is suddenly giving you pain.

Migraineurs report that the following things sometimes trigger migraines:

- Bright lights
- Cigarette or cigar smoke
- Environmental changes (weather, heat, cold)
- Fatigue or hangover
- Menopause or perimenopause
- Menstrual cycle
- Puberty
- Sexual activity
- Sleep disturbances (restlessness, insomnia)
- Sleep patterns (uneven sleeping, getting up and going to bed at different times, and a wide range in the number of hours you sleep)
- Smells and sounds
- Surgery/anesthesia
- Travel
- Worries, anxiety, stress

Most people have triggers. For you, the question is "How many of these triggers have to team up in order to cause a migraine?" You may tiptoe past triggers all the time, and they don't make themselves known as bugaboos as long as you're still hovering below your threshold. Your head gets a full frontal attack only when your body's forces get overwhelmed by enemies packing enormous pain bolts. In other words, it often takes a village of triggers to raise a headache.

Stopping Triggers in Their Tracks

Several lifestyle issues can influence the severity and frequency of your headaches. Make sure you follow these guidelines:

- ✔ **Stay far, far away from red wine, aged cheeses (especially sharp Cheddar), and caffeinated coffee.** Caffeinated coffee is a problem because trying to go cold turkey when kicking caffeine can give you withdrawal headaches, and if you're predisposed to migraines, you can bet that your headaches will be killer. Taper off caffeine intake over a period of a week or so.

- ✔ **Don't smoke.**

- ✔ **Get plenty of rest.** Don't sleep 12 hours a night, but don't get exhausted to the gills, either. The right amount of rest varies with each individual; you can often tell what your body requires by checking the number of hours you sleep naturally, when no alarm or person wakes you up. For some people, it may be six hours — for others, it may be eight or nine.

✔ **Bump up the fiber content of your diet.** Eat more whole-grain cereals and breads, and more veggies.

✔ **Eat very few fat- or sugar-laden foods.**

✔ **Get enough calcium and magnesium.** Every day, you need about 1,200 mg of calcium and 300 mg of magnesium. (If your diet is deficient in these, you can use vitamin supplements.) Doctors see low magnesium levels in women who are on birth control pills, are having PMS symptoms, or are taking estrogen-only hormone replacement for menopause. Studies show a link between low magnesium and migraines in women *and* men. Some researchers even go so far as to suggest that the root of all migraine evil is a deficiency of magnesium.

✔ **Avoid migraine triggers such as alcohol, chocolate, artificial sweeteners, concentrated sugar, pickled foods, MSG, cured meats (with nitrates), sulfites, olives, snow peas, and pickles.** Sulfites are found in maraschino cherries, instant potatoes, frozen French fries, shredded coconut, dried fruits, syrups, soup mixes, vegetable juices, fruit juices, lemon juice, wine, raisins, and pizza. MSG is often in Chinese foods, processed meats, tenderizers, canned and processed foods, and soy sauce.

✔ **Laugh.**

✔ **Meditate.**

✔ **Walk or work out regularly.** But don't turn into a workout fanatic. Over-exercising can decrease estrogen. As with everything, try the moderation route. (And be sure to warm up before workouts.)

Triggers get together and party hearty

Here's how triggers wreak havoc:

Let's say that you know alcohol always gives you a headache, but one night at a friend's wedding reception, you just can't resist a glass of Champagne. (You're dying to be "normal," so you make a toast and chug-a-lug the bubbly.)

Ah-hah! No migraine! *Whoa!* You're impressed. This is a sign. An omen. It must mean that you've finally outgrown that irksome alcohol trigger altogether, right? Wrong.

What it means is that when wine, Champagne, or a mixed drink gave you a headache in the past, the drink had some partners in crime. You drank it on a day when other factors were working their black magic — you were about to start your menstrual period, you just finished a 12-hour workday, or you skipped lunch. Or all three.

Judiciously avoiding food triggers is one of the smartest things a migraine sufferer can do to help herself.

Instead of drinking alcohol when you know you'll be sorry you did, drown your disappointment in white wedding cake or cute groomsmen (or bridesmaids).

Chapter 3

Distinguishing a Migraine from Other Head Pain

* *

In This Chapter

▶ Developing a better understanding of migraines

▶ Recognizing variations on migraines

▶ Preventing rebound headaches

▶ Debunking common myths

* *

To fight the good fight, you must know your enemy. The biggest problem with headache-sorting is that people mistakenly think that they have migraines when their headaches are of a different type, or they don't think that they have migraines when they actually do. It's a wild, wild world out there in Headache Land, and figuring out your skull signals is the first step to taming your migraine headaches.

This chapter helps you get up close and personal with different types of headaches to find out whether you have bona-fide migraines. We clue you in to symptoms of the various types of headaches.

By the time you're through with this chapter, you'll be madly conversant in headache-speak and amazingly savvy about the headache universe.

To get in on the New Day of Migraine Management, you need to first look at the different types of headaches and the physiological path of migraines. This information paves your way to the next step — getting your doctor's help in figuring out whether your head pain fits the migraine mold or is the result of another type of headache or health condition. After you determine what is causing your headaches, you'll be ready to zero in on the best treatments.

Ranking Primary and Secondary Headaches

Generally speaking, headaches fall into two categories: primary (the headache as the problem) and secondary (the headache as a symptom of an organic disease). With *primary headaches,* the headache itself is the big, bad Goliath causing your symptoms. When you have a primary migraine headache, you can't blame anything but the alpha dog — the migraine. Migraines are primary headaches. With *secondary headaches,* the headache is one of the symptoms caused by another medical condition. A headache caused by meningitis is an example of a secondary headache.

Headaches are also categorized as either episodic or chronic. *Episodic headaches* are headaches that you have now and then. Headaches are considered *chronic headaches* if you have them for more than

15 days per month. The conventional wisdom suggests that most chronic headaches stem from sinus disease, eye problems, or allergies. The fact is that most people who suffer from chronic headaches have migraine or tension-type headaches — and few of these folks have other health problems that contribute to their headaches.

Headaches can be especially hard to diagnose, because they often have conflicting symptoms. The following traits show the chameleon nature of headaches:

✔ Headaches can mutate from one type to another.

✔ You may suffer from more than one type of headache.

✔ Your headache type may fit into two categories at the same time.

All of these traits can apply to migraines as well as to other types of headaches.

Spotting Migraine Impersonators

Because many people automatically think that a bad headache is a migraine, it's easy for all types of headaches to be mistakenly labeled migraines. This confusion can be dangerous if you have a brain hemorrhage and you treat it as though it's a migraine. The improper treatment can result in a potentially fatal delay in getting help.

Another danger in treating a headache as though it's a migraine is that you may take the wrong medication. Some drugs are headache-specific. In other words, certain medications work best on cluster headaches, some target tension-type headaches, and others are migraine-specific (see Chapter 5 for more on migraine medications).

Ah, clearly a migraine by any other name would still be . . . yes, a migraine. But headaches can only be considered migraines if they come with the unique characteristics of migrainehood. You need to get acquainted with the head bangers that only masquerade in the guise of the Big M, but are really cluster or tension-type renegades. Their symptoms are no picnic, mind you, but these migraine impersonators shouldn't be mistaken for a true migraine.

If you have bad headaches that aren't migraines, you may have tension-type headaches or, much less likely, cluster headaches (see the following sections).

The following headache characteristics are signals that you probably don't have a migraine:

- ✔ Your pain is a dull ache without any throbbing.

- ✔ Your shoulders and neck muscles feel knotted-up.

- ✔ You get a headache only after exercise or sex.

- ✔ Your headaches are getting steadily worse. *Warning:* This symptom may be a sign of an *organic headache* — a headache caused by a problem such as an abnormality in the brain or skull. An abnormality may be a brain aneurysm, a brain tumor, a hematoma, meningitis, a brain infection or abscess, encephalitis, or a cerebral hemorrhage.

Encapsulating the cluster headache

By looking at the traits of the other headaches that may be mistaken for migraines, you can detect the differences and key into the type that you actually have. For example, cluster headaches, which are often even more painful than migraines, are rare. They frequently occur at night, and they target men more often than women. The following symptoms can indicate a cluster headache:

- ✔ **You have a sudden, piercing pain on one side of your head.**

- ✔ **You have a cluster of symptoms.** You may have pain behind one eye on one side of your head; your eye (on the pain side) may become red and tear up; your eyelid may droop; and your nostril on the pain side may feel congested or runny.

- ✔ **You have several headaches per day over a period of weeks or months.** Because headache attacks group up, the word *cluster* is used to describe them.

- ✔ **Your headaches last 30 to 90 minutes (or a few hours).**

Some researchers contend that cluster headaches reflect a dysfunction of your brain's *hypothalamus* (the portion of the brain that secretes substances that control various body functions). Another hypothesis is that your neck arteries are feeding incorrect amounts of oxygen and carbon dioxide to your brain by way of your blood.

Cluster headaches respond well to medication. Another popular treatment is oxygen therapy, where you're zapped with oxygen through a facemask. The oxygen can get rid of your pain if the treatment takes place early in an attack.

Cluster headaches can be like stormy rain clouds. They move around, they sprinkle darkness here and there, and they show up now and then. Your headache goes away and then pops up again later the same day. Some people report having as many as eight headaches in a single day!

One type of headache similar to cluster headaches is chronic paroxysmal hemicrania. Lasting about 10 to 20 minutes, this headache has a tendency to come and go many times in a given day. *Paroxysms* refer to stabbing pains happening in rapid succession, usually around the eye area. *Hemicranial* means "half of the head," or a one-sided pain. Combine the two and you have stabbing pains on one side of the head that are chronic (experienced periodically over a long period of time). About half of the people with severe migraines have one-sided pain, but if you have this symptom with chronic paroxysmal hemicrania, it's likely that a doctor will recommend an MRI, because it can be a sign that a tumor or abnormal blood vessel is causing your headaches. If you have chronic paroxysmal hemicrania, you may have this type of headache off and on for several years.

Untangling tension-type headaches

Tension-type headaches are as common as dirt. These headaches are the kind that anyone can experience at pretty much any time. You feel the pain, all right, but tension-type headaches typically respond fairly quickly to pain medication — ibuprofen or acetaminophen — or physical therapy, such as neck and shoulder exercises or massage.

For some tension-type headache sufferers, learning better stress-handling techniques and eliminating triggers can help alleviate their headaches.

When tension-type headaches are episodic (occurring randomly), they can usually be relieved with over-the-counter (OTC) medications. But if you take medication almost daily for your headaches, see a doctor, because you're probably having chronic tension-type headaches. (Your headaches may be chronic if you're having them most days, and the trend has been in place for months.)

You may get a tension-type headache because you tense up when you're under stress — if this is the case, your headache stems from muscle tension. Or you may get tension-type headaches when you're hungry or exhausted.

The following conditions are suspected causes of chronic tension-type headaches:

- ✔ Abnormalities in the brain's pain control system
- ✔ Abnormalities of the neck muscles, bones, or jaw
- ✔ Depression
- ✔ Emotional factors, such as worry, dread, fear, and excitement
- ✔ Eyestrain
- ✔ Fatigue
- ✔ Misaligned teeth
- ✔ Poor posture
- ✔ Stress

Don't be confused by the word *tension*. Tension isn't always the cause of this type of headache.

If your headaches are the tension-type, you have some of the following symptoms:

- ✔ Your skull feels tender, and your headache can be characterized as a dull, constant ache that's mild or moderate on the pain scale.

- ✔ You feel a pressure or bandlike sensation around the upper area of both sides of your head (as if you're wearing a headband that's five sizes too small), or the back of your head hurts.

- ✔ Your neck and shoulder muscles feel tightly knotted.

- ✔ You don't vomit, get nauseated, or have visual disturbances (in contrast to some migraines).

- ✔ The pain creeps up slowly.

Usually, you get these headaches during times of high stress, but you may also have the same type of headache on a day without stress.

If you have tension-type headaches all the time (the kind that people call "sick headaches"), you may be the unlucky recipient of the dynamic duo — coexisting migraine and tension-type headaches. This combination is also called a *transformed migraine*. The tension/migraine pairing comes with varied symptoms that befit its hybrid nature. People who have coexisting migraine and tension-type headaches often overuse medications because they experience day-to-day head pain. The overuse of medication can induce rebounding problems (see "Recoiling from Rebound Headaches," later in this chapter) and cause individual migraine attacks to evolve into chronic daily headaches.

Understanding What Makes a Migraine a Migraine

A good starting point is defining what a migraine actually is — an issue that undoubtedly flips through your mind once or twice when you're lying on your bed, grasping your head, wondering what this madness is all about.

First, you need to understand that a migraine isn't just a headache. Oh, no. It's a headache and more — or the more without the headache.

Headaches aren't the only symptom of migraines. Migraines are an umbrella for multiple symptoms, one of which is the headache (and even the headaches come in a wide range of painfulness).

Basically, if you have throbbing head pain along with three (or more) of the following symptoms, you probably have migraines:

✔ Auras (visual disturbances, such as flashing lights, that precede the headache)

✔ Sensitivity to light, smells, and sounds

✔ Stomach problems, such as nausea, vomiting, or diarrhea

✔ A drooping eyelid

✔ A pale face or a flushed or very red face or a face that's extra sensitive

✔ A tender scalp

✔ Bloodshot eyes

✔ Blurred vision

✔ Cold hands and feet, or a feeling of being hot all over

✔ Dizziness or a feeling of spinning

✔ Food cravings or a total loss of appetite

Note: Most people have migraines without auras, but some do experience migraines with auras.

Migraine headaches are intermittent — once a week, perhaps, or once a month or year; you don't have them every day. However, a single headache can last for days.

Some migraine symptoms are also indicative of other medical conditions, such as stroke or seizure. So you need to see your doctor to confirm the diagnosis of migraine.

Because everyone's migraines are a bit different, your reality may be some combination of common migraine symptoms, but you can generally expect symptoms similar to the following:

✔ Pain affects one side of the head, is moderate to severe to almost unbearable, can be described as "throbbing" or "hammering," and may last two hours to three days or more.

✔ Stomach symptoms include lack of appetite, stomach pain, nausea or vomiting (after which you feel better), constipation and/or diarrhea.

✔ Sensory symptoms include sensitivity to light, noise, or smells; visual disturbances (zigzagging or flashing lights, or partial vision) that precede your head pain.

✔ Symptoms in your limbs include weakness in an arm or leg, or both; tingling and/or numbness in your arms and face; and cold hands and feet.

You may also feel disoriented or dizzy, and you may experience mood changes — you feel unusually lethargic and "down."

Tracking the stages of a migraine

Rarely is a migraine as simple as "just the headache pain." Sometimes it *is* just that — no more, no less. Often, though, migraines come with other symptoms (see the previous section). Your symptoms may usher you through some or all of the phases/stages described in the following list:

- ✔ **Prodrome:** This stage may occur anytime from a few hours to two days before a headache begins. You may feel an extraordinary sensitivity to lights, sounds, and smells. Your mood may be gloomy or blue, although some people are downright euphoric during this stage. Many people yawn. Your hands and feet may feel cold.

- ✔ **Aura:** Some migraine sufferers have this stage, but most don't. The aura usually amounts to a brief period (15 to 45 minutes) of visual disturbances. Less common symptoms include numbness, weakness, or even changes in the way you see things.

- ✔ **Headache:** This phase can last anywhere from two hours to three days (the duration of migraines varies greatly). The Big Kahuna Migraine pitches a tent in your head to stay for a while — this can be painful, nauseating, dizzying, and more. The onset of the pain is usually gradual. The pain may be felt on one or both sides of your head, or it may change sides during your headache.

✔ **Recovery and postdrome:** The headache finally fades, leaving you in a bummed-out slump during which you feel like you've been drawn and quartered. The postdrome phase typically lasts about a day. During this phase, you may feel physically worthless. On the other hand, some folks in postdrome move into a full-tilt energy phase, totally high on life because they're finally free of the pain. Some even experience a truly euphoric day of huge productivity, much like the mood that is sometimes seen in prodrome.

Figure 3-1 charts the whole process.

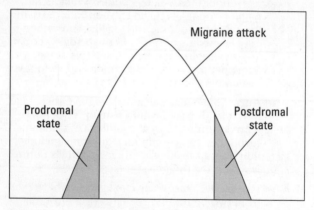

Figure 3-1: Charting the course of a migraine.

Tracing the trek through your brain

Investigators believe that you can blame the symptoms of migraine — from pain to vomiting to aura — on specific brain-related changes. The blood vessels, by the way, are viewed as the supporting actors in the grand drama of the migraine, while the nerve cells appear to be the rabble-rousers.

Getting inside your head for a closer look

Today's high-tech imaging equipment thrills researchers! With help from some very cool imaging equipment, they can get inside the heads of migraine sufferers and actually watch what happens in the brain when a migraine attack occurs.

The ability to view the brain during a migraine attack has helped clarify the migraine mechanism somewhat. Researchers have noted that the brain's neurons are more hyperactive than normal during migraine headaches. And it appears that the activity shoots down from the top of the brain to the brain stem, where key pain centers are found. In people who have migraines (but not other types of headache), this rampant electrical feistiness takes place in the brain stem. So some researchers have concluded that migraine pain either springs from the revving up of these pain centers in the brain stem or from the blood vessels and nerves around the brain getting stimulated from spreading excitation.

The migraine aura is believed to be due to a wave of electrical excitation that moves across the surface of the brain. It is followed by the depression of electrical activity. The electrical activity can activate pain nerves and start the migraine headache.

You have to figure one more fact into the equation: The migraine sufferer must be exposed to triggers (or just one trigger) — a combination of menstrual hormones, a specific type of food, and high anxiety, for example — that set the fright-night headache in motion.

Well, even if you don't care about the scoop on the birth of a migraine, or you don't think that it makes much sense, all you really need is a general idea of the thrashing-about that's going on in your brain in order to understand why the chaos can make your head hurt.

Researchers think that migraine headaches come from a disturbed blood flow to the brain that results when arteries first narrow and then swell. The *vascular theory* — that a migraine results from the expansion of blood vessels in the brain — is no longer believed. Many migraine-treatment medications that constrict dilated vessels have effects on systems beyond blood circulation.

Scientists had long noted that migraine pain occurred when blood vessels on the surface of the brain dilated, but *why* they dilated was less of an issue. As it turns out, these headaches originate in the brain stem, and the pain arises from changes in brain chemistry. The prevalent belief now is that the migraine-prone person gets exposed to a trigger (or triggers), and then brain cells emit chemicals that cause the expansion of blood vessels on the surface of the brain. The vessels, upon widening, stimulate nerve fibers, thus resulting in throbbing pain.

The head honchos on headaches (the people who do headache research and study scientific evidence) contend that problems with the brain's *neurotransmitters* (brain-messenger chemicals) are the real villains behind migraine and tension-type headaches, which were previously (and erroneously) called muscle-contraction headaches. Communication between the neurotransmitters and brain cells (neurons) breaks down, and the levels of serotonin and other brain-messenger chemicals fluctuate — a big problem for your body, because serotonin plays a role in your ability to feel pain. Therefore, when migraineurs take medications that affect their serotonin levels, many of them get better fast. (See Chapter 5 for medications.)

Migraines are generated in the brain stem. When pain centers of the brain stem get revved up, the spreading excitation appears to stimulate blood vessels and nerves in the brain. Thus, a migraine can occur when a person has a genetic tendency and certain neurochemical changes take place in the brain, leading to a spiral that results in the brain doing quirky chemical cartwheels that spur a vascular process. Why? The chemical brain messengers are thrown off balance, which irritates the blood vessels and thus alters blood flow to the brain. After this occurs, pain signals are sent back to the brain stem.

Identifying Variations on the Migraine Theme

As if migraines aren't big enough mischief-makers as it is, they also like to sing show tunes and take on different personas. So here we turn to *migraine variants* — the exceptions and odd lots that make finding your way to migraine diagnosis and treatment quite a challenging proposition.

Abdominal migraines

Abdominal migraines, which are sometimes diagnosed in children, are unusual because they cause pain in the stomach and lead to nausea and vomiting (sometimes without a headache).

A child who complains of recurrent pain in his stomach may be experiencing abdominal migraines. Children who suffer from abdominal migraines are likely to have migraine headaches in adulthood. Abdominal migraines are usually treated with anticonvulsant drugs.

Basilar migraines

The basilar migraine was once known as the basilar artery migraine, or BAM. It was considered to be a problem that was found primarily in young women and adolescent girls, but it occurs in both sexes and all ages. Basilar migraines are extremely rare, but they have the potential to be a serious health hazard in that they can lead to a transient ischemic attack (TIA) or stroke.

Symptoms to watch for are double vision, partial vision loss, terrible vomiting, dizziness, loss of balance, slurred speech, lack of coordination, numbness (on one or both sides of the body), weakness, and confusion. These symptoms typically go away at the onset of the actual headache, although they may last for days after the pain disappears.

If you experience any of the symptoms that signal basilar migraines, see a doctor as soon as possible.

Transient ischemic attacks, which can result from basilar migraines (although they rarely do), are essentially "mini-strokes." TIAs result from disruptions of the blood flow to the brain. Although a stroke can mean permanent disability, TIAs don't cause lasting damage. Any neurologic problems associated with TIAs, such as weakness in one arm and slurred speech, are resolved within 24 hours.

Hemiplegic migraines

Hemiplegic migraines are often caused by an inherited gene, but they occur in people with no family history of migraines. With hemiplegic migraines, you experience temporary paralysis or arm and leg weakness on one side of your body. The paralysis or weakness is then followed, usually within an hour, by bad head pain. The paralysis or weakness does not always go away when the headache disappears. These headaches often originate during childhood.

Ocular migraines

Ocular migraines are rare migraines that feature a repeated vision disturbance (temporary, partial, or complete vision loss in one eye) that lasts less than one hour. After the vision disturbance subsides, you're left with a dull ache behind the affected eye, and your entire head may ache, as well.

If you suffer from ocular migraines, you need to be evaluated by a doctor (an ophthalmologist) to exclude other possible causes for your vision loss.

Ophthalmoplegic migraines

Ophthalmoplegic migraines are no longer believed to be migraines. They are now thought to be a type of *neuritis* (inflammation of a nerve). These headaches are associated with pain around the eyeball and the temporary weakness or paralysis of eye muscle(s). It's a condition that's usually diagnosed in children. The common symptoms of these migraines are a drooping eyelid, a dilated pupil, and double vision.

Ophthalmoplegic migraines, which can last for days or months, require a thorough exam and testing to rule out conditions that are more serious.

Status migrainosus

The term *status migrainosus* refers to a migraine attack that goes on for more than 72 hours and leads to problems such as dehydration.

 If you have status migrainosus, you should go to the emergency room, where you will be treated with IV fluids and pain medication.

Women-only migraines

Certain migraines are uniquely attached to the hormonal swings that females experience. Migraines are commonly linked to menstruation. Some women get migraine headaches when they're on oral contraceptives. And in the case of women who are going through or are past menopause, hormone therapy migraines can be problematic. (Some older women have hormone-replacement-therapy-related headaches, while other women who have had migraines in the past no longer have them after menopause.)

Recoiling from Rebound Headaches

A *rebound headache* is a headache that you end up with just because you go in search of a little relief from the constant pounding in your noggin. You feel bad, so you take a pill — you feel worse, so you take another, and so on, and so on, and scoobie-doobie-do.

Basically, you wind up with a headache because you're overusing medications.

 Exceeding label or physician instructions when taking medications can result in rebounding into another headache. Other spin-offs of medication overuse include a more excruciatingly painful headache, addiction to medications, and other adverse side effects. Prolonged use of even over-the-counter medicines can cause liver and kidney damage.

In the wild-and-woolly migraine arena, rebound headaches have to rank right up there at the top of the pain-wielding, mind-blowing, frustration-inciting extravaganza. Sometimes rebound headaches are migraines, and sometimes they're not.

To help prevent future rebound headaches, you may be able to take a migraine-preventive medication or use lifestyle changes without medication. First, however, you must get past the vicious cycle of rebounding — you overmedicate over and over before realizing that you're perpetuating your pain. Your doctor can help you taper off your overmedicating, nonproductive ways.

If some of the following signs apply to you, you're probably having rebound headaches (but be sure to see your doctor for evaluation of your problem to confirm that it's a headache and not something more serious):

✔ You suffer from headaches daily or every other day.

✔ Your pain intensifies about three hours after your last dose of medication.

✔ Your pain medications don't work as well as they used to.

✔ You take more medication, but your headaches are worse.

✔ You rely on more pills, and you take them more often.

✔ You take medication even for mild headaches, and you often try to ward off a headache by using a medication.

✔ You take pain relievers three to four days a week, and you average more than three tablets per day. (This depends on the kind of medication you're taking, so you'll need your doctor's advice.)

✔ Your pain runs the gamut from mild to moderate to horrible. Usually, the pain is a dull ache that you feel on both sides of your forehead and, sometimes, on the top or back of your head.

✔ Your headaches occur much more frequently.

Because you're in pain, you may use medications too often. The theory behind the rebound headache is that the overuse of drugs makes the headache rebound after your body has absorbed all of the medication. Painkillers are supposed to relieve pain, of course, but if you overuse prescription or nonprescription drugs, they can turn on you and actually cause headaches.

Essentially, an over-the-counter drug or a prescription medication that's taken too often can give rise to a brain-craving for more of the medicine. The episode begins when the brain gets some initial relief from pain, likes the effect, and then decides it will send out to room service for more of the same. Your brain continues to signal "pain" in its search for more of the drug, and you have to take increasing dosages to get relief. Therefore, your medication becomes less and less effective, and you create a cycle of increasing misery.

If you rush to the emergency room with a killer migraine, the doctor will want to know what you took and when you took it last, so be prepared to supply this information. The emergency room physician needs to know if you overused medication and have a rebound headache. She doesn't want to treat you with a medication you overused, or with a medication that's not going to jibe with a drug you took recently.

The typical medications that appear in the rebound scenario are aspirin and aceta-minophen, alone or in combination with caffeine-containing products. Other drug culprits often implicated in rebounding are

- ✔ Caffeine
- ✔ Codeine
- ✔ Combination drugs such as Fiorinal and Midrin
- ✔ Drugs containing barbiturates
- ✔ Ergotamine tartrate
- ✔ Opiates

Abortive drugs (such as the nonsteroidals ibuprofen and naproxen), triptans (Imitrex, Zomig, Amerge), and DHE (dihydroergotamine) may also induce rebound-ing, but they're less likely to do so.

For more details about medications, see Chapters 4 and 5.

Knowing what can make you feel worse

Rebound headaches occur innocently enough: You feel a headache coming on, so you take an over-the-counter pain reliever, such as ibuprofen, aspirin, or acetaminophen, or a prescription medication, such as the oft-prescribed Midrin. Ordinarily, the drug you take works well, and you use it on an occasional basis. This time, however, you don't get relief soon enough. So you take the daily recommended dose (or more) three times during one week, and the result is a rebound headache that's worse and longer-lasting than the one you had to begin with.

Another route for getting a rebound is trying to stave off a headache — because you remember how painful your last migraine was, you begin taking medication at the first hint of a headache.

 As a rule, you risk a rebound headache if you take pain relievers for more than two days in a row, in a seven-day period. Depending on the particular medication, taking even one or two pills of a prescription medication per day is enough to result in a rebound headache in many people, but it's more typical for someone to take more than one or two tablets.

The phrase *analgesic rebound headache* refers specifically to the excessive use of pain relievers — a major factor in the transformation of episodic migraine into chronic daily headache, often called *transformed migraine.*

An analgesic is basically a pain-relief medication. Non-narcotic analgesics such as acetaminophen (Tylenol) are used to treat mild- to medium-pain migraines. Some analgesic products contain caffeine as an added ingredient to help pump up the pain-killing impact.

A few too many OTC drugs — and, ay, carumba! What a headache!

We know a New York–based flight attendant who was taking OTC drugs to self-treat her headaches. She had not been diagnosed with migraines, but she thought that her headaches resembled the migraines her mother had always experienced.

"Everybody's taking something for headaches, and I was definitely gulping a lot of pills. Finally, as it turned out, my episodic headaches were transformed into chronic daily headaches, or that's how the ER doctor explained it when my fiancé took me to the emergency room. I was lying down in the car, and my head was splitting — I really, truly thought I was dying. The doctor had me see a headache specialist, who told me I'd had a rebound or drug-induced headache. He said that both over-the-counter and prescription meds can cause rebounding if they're taken too often."

Looking back, she is glad that her "crisis" led her to get help — something she should have done years earlier. "My doctor told me that I wouldn't have gotten better on my own, and that rebounding can be very painful and troublesome. He took me off these drugs, and it was two months before I finally quit having frequent headaches. Then, he helped me come up with a treatment plan that was much healthier and targeted my migraines better."

Overusing OTC medications that contain caffeine often leads to rebound headaches. Consider the fact that some of these tablets contain up to 60 mg of caffeine per pill. Therefore, if you take ten tablets a day — not extraordinary for a migraine sufferer — you get quite a major pile-up of caffeine.

Adding to the risk of rebound headaches is excessive caffeine consumption. If you drink four or more cups of coffee (or six colas or cups of tea) a day, you may have trouble.

 You may also get rebound headaches or weekend migraines when you fail to consume your usual amount of caffeine. If you normally drink seven cups of coffee at work, Monday through Friday, and then you drop down to one cup on Saturday, the drastic plummet in caffeine intake can give your body a jolt. The drop in caffeine may cause your blood vessels to widen and lead to a migraine. This example drives home a fact that many migraine sufferers have discovered the hard way — you can't drink five cups of coffee and other caffeinated drinks per day and then suddenly just cut yourself off, unless you want to suffer a mammoth headache.

Desperate but dumb

We heard about a guy whose everlasting headache pushed him over the edge of the abyss into a horrible pain place. He thought that his migraine was going to last forever. He had it for six days, and he kept taking one medication after another, but nothing helped.

Finally, he took some pills that his housemate used to help relieve a headache he had after a surgical procedure. After a day of dosing with his housemate's pills, he was suspended in a terrible headache. Feeling very panicky, he called his doctor, who had him stop taking both kinds of medications and try some ways to get pain relief without drugs. After two days of relaxation techniques and head massages, he finally rejoined the land of the living.

To cut back on your intake of caffeine, use a tapering-off approach. Start by cutting down slightly on coffee, cola, chocolate, and tea, and keep reducing your consumption by 6 ounces each week. Also, reduce your use of caffeine-containing medication. To avoid a withdrawal headache, stay at each new intake level for several days. If possible, set your sights on a caffeine-free diet, which is ideal for your overall health and your avoidance of migraines.

Getting off the rebound treadmill

What's the answer for rebound headaches? Stop taking the medications that are causing you trouble. In the case of nonprescription drugs, stop taking them immediately, or taper off over two to three days.

If you have questions about how to taper off your offending medication, or if you're still hurting from the vicious circle-pain-rebound migraine, call your doctor for advice. Your doctor may start you on a preventive medication, but it won't be very effective until you discontinue using the overused medication and it's out of your system. (The length of time that drugs stay in your system varies greatly, depending on the drug, so you need to rely on your doctor's advice when discontinuing the use of a drug.)

During your withdrawal from the offending medication(s), which can take several weeks, your headaches get worse before they get better. Within a few hours after you stop taking the drugs, your head begins to hurt even more, and the pain continues to gain momentum for a day or two. Have your doctor monitor your progress and, if necessary, give you a transition dose of a medication that you can use temporarily to get past the rough spots.

Hospitalization may be necessary if you're discontinuing the long-term use of ergotamine or
narcotics (opiates). You must detox from these
medications to reduce migraine frequency and free
up your system to be responsive to preventives.

Naturally, you may feel oh so stupid and silly for perpetuating your own headache by taking too many pills, but
don't think that it's just you — most migraine sufferers
do this at some point. When you're caught in a pain
trap and you can't get out, you try almost anything —
and that's how you got on the rebound merry-go-round
in the first place. Just make a point of etching firmly in
your mind how very awful a rebound headache can be.
This thought will slap down your hand the next time
you're a bit hasty in reaching for your pain medications.

This cycle of dependency is both frightening and hard
to handle. Sometimes the only solution is to slap an
ice pack or cooling pad on your head and ride it out
cold turkey. (Repeat a positive affirmation: "This will
spiral to an end at some point. Within 24 hours — this
time tomorrow — the pain will be gone.")

 Biofeedback and behavioral therapy are sometimes used to treat mood disturbances that are
occasionally associated with chronic daily
headaches.

Typically, people who work on reducing their dependency on medications after experiencing the rebound
crucible eventually reach a plateau where they have
migraines less often, and the migraines aren't as bad
as previous ones. In most cases of rebound, the long-
term outcome is very promising. Moreover, you don't
have to fear another rebound skirmish, because your
doctor can provide you with an improved treatment
plan for future migraines.

Defusing the Myths

Migraines often go undiagnosed for years. Many people flounder around with the pain and other symptoms and fail to get proper solutions because they're trapped in the migraine myths, such as "What you have isn't a migraine, because my brother has them, and he always throws up, and you don't" or "People who have migraines are always depressed."

Despite myths to the contrary, migraines are real and valid physical problems that require concrete solutions. Your migraine probably carries a whole constellation of sidekick symptoms that need to be addressed. In other words, pulling yourself up by your bootstraps just won't do it. Don't let anyone tell you that the pain is "all in your head." It's not! Hard-throbbing head pain is certainly not the stuff fantasies are made of.

Some folks think that they know exactly what constitutes a migraine; other folks only know what migraines aren't. Table 3-1 lays out some of the common myths and realities of migraines.

Table 3-1   Migraine Myths and Realities

Myth	Reality
Migraines have certain, specific symptoms that make them migraines, and if your headaches are at all different, they're not migraines.	There are a multitude of migraine symptoms, of which one symptom or a combination of symptoms indicates a true migraine.

(continued)

Table 3-1 *(continued)*

Myth	Reality
All migraineurs have the same symptoms.	Migraineurs experience different symptoms. Migraines are very individualistic. Your migraines may be totally different from those of another migraine sufferer you happen to know.
Migraines are psychological, not physiological.	Migraines are definitely physiological in nature, causing distinct neurological changes. They're not just "in your head."
Your doctor is completely familiar with all migraine symptoms and should be able to diagnose you just by hearing that you have headaches sometimes.	Some doctors are more adept at headache diagnosis than others. But even the most skilled diagnostician will need you to provide a clear picture of your headaches to aid him in diagnosing your head pain.

If you want your physician to have your treasure-trove of personal health history at his fingertips, you must be good at info-sharing. So if you tell your family doctor that you have occasional headaches that are killers, but you fail to flesh out the symptoms, your physician won't have enough information to help you. Be as specific as possible.

You have to be your number-one advocate in health-care delivery. You should know your body better than anyone else; you should be quite familiar with your existing health conditions and the medications you take. You're definitely a pro at describing what's troubling you. Your valuable input allows you and your physician to cut through myths and misconceptions and get to the truth.

No, she wasn't going crazy

No, you're not imagining things or trying to creep people out when you say that your head hurts like crazy. So will someone please listen?

Sometimes it's super-difficult to get headaches diagnosed correctly. You may feel a little goony just having them, and you really hate getting into all the gruesome details. Or you're afraid that when you try to bring up the subject, your doctor will think that you're some whining little hypochondriac, or that you're wildly exaggerating. Sound familiar?

A Houston postal worker had headaches so debilitating that she was missing work often. The situation scared her because, as a single mom, she was the only wage-earner in the family, and it was her job to "bring home the bacon and fry it up in a pan." What if she got fired for missing so much work?

Soft-spoken and undemanding, this woman mentioned her headaches to her gynecologist, who patted her hand and told her that she was under a lot of stress as a single mother. He didn't ask about other symptoms, and she didn't volunteer any information. But the truth was, bright lights made her headaches worse, and over-the-counter meds never helped. Plus, she felt nauseated every time a headache hit, which was invariably right around the time she began her period each month.

One day, she casually unloaded her symptoms on a customer who was writing a book on migraines (and buying stamps). The writer told her that the symptoms sounded like a migraine. But she said, "No, my doctor didn't diagnose me with migraines."

There's the rub. Who knows more about your own hurting head than you? Try to convey all of your symptoms to your doctor, because one thing is for sure — he won't be able to guess them!

Chapter 4

Spelling Relief without a Prescription

. . . .

In This Chapter

▶ Trying over-the-counter pills

▶ Sidestepping the mistake of overusing over-the-counter drugs

▶ Using vitamin and herbal supplements to fight migraines

. . . .

*Y*ou have a quandary on your hands: You hate headaches, but you don't like taking prescription drugs. This aversion to drugs is just a personal quirk of yours, but it's a very real concern for you in your search for headache relief.

So, in your crusade to curb migraine pain, you look at non-prescription options, starting with first-tier headache medications — the over-the-counter drugs you buy at the drugstore or grocery store. Of course, you can't expect over-the-counter medications to pack the same kind of wallop as a heavy-duty pre-scription medication, but sometimes a little dab will do you.

You may want to go over the counter at your whole-foods/health store and stock up on herbal and vitamin remedies.

In this chapter, we talk about the pros and cons of non-prescription treatments that may be just what the doctor ordered . . . so to speak.

Counting on Over-the-Counter Medications

Some folks just hate prescription drugs. They don't like the way certain drugs made them feel in the past. If you belong to this school of thought, you may be drawn to a less aggressive, over-the-counter (OTC) approach to pain-fighting.

Generally thought of as kinder and gentler than prescription medications, OTC remedies include ibuprofen and acetaminophen, which can usually knock out a relatively mild migraine. Aspirin typically isn't strong enough to provide relief for migraines. (Advil, Excedrin, and Motrin are popular over-the-counter headache relievers.)

Even if you're not adverse to taking prescription drugs, try OTCs first, because they're less apt to sideline you. With OTCs, you're probably not going to get drowsy or woozy to the point where you're unable to work, drive, or cope with your kids.

If you're a migraineur who gets relief from OTC medications, good for you. But don't feel discouraged or turn cranky if OTC medications don't do the trick for you. You may need a prescription pain reliever for those times when you experience a truly difficult headache, and that's nothing to be ashamed of.

Comparing benefits

If you have severe migraines, it's pretty unlikely that a medication you can buy over the counter will provide the kind of pain relief you need. But that doesn't mean that you can't try OTC medications — exceptions to every rule do exist. If you prefer to try OTC medications first, you definitely should.

People may tell you otherwise, but it's actually possible for some migraine sufferers to overcome their pain without prescription medication. According to the National Headache Foundation Web site (www. headaches.org), about 60 percent of migraine sufferers use OTC remedies exclusively to manage their headaches.

Sometimes OTC remedies fail to provide you with any type of relief. Other times, they may provide you with a little relief — enough to help you handle the discomfort until your headache is completely resolved with sleep or another dose of the medicine later in the day. If you're one of the lucky ones, you may even find an OTC drug that works very well almost every time you get a headache.

But if your headache is "killing" you, and OTC pills aren't helping, OTC remedies will seem about as effective as tying a banana peel to your forehead (a custom, in some cultures, that produces a cool look but is worthless as pain relief).

By the way, if you take an OTC tablet referred to as a "migraine formula," don't think that you're practically taking a prescription drug. The truth is that migraine formulas are no stronger than their sibling over-the-counter medications. The U.S. Food and Drug Administration (FDA) allows drug companies to label their products as migraine formulas even though they often don't provide any extra benefits for migraine sufferers.

Take OTC pain meds early in your migraine attack, but don't take them often. Don't exceed recommended dosages!

If you take OTC pills for more than two days each week, you may make your pain situation worse. Unfortunately, you may have to wait two or three hours for an OTC drug to relieve your pain. This delay may tempt you to pop more pills in hopes of a quicker resolution. But you must avoid the trap of taking OTC drugs too often; if you're not careful, you may experience increased side effects (stomach upset) or get a rebound headache, which can evolve into a very painful problem (see Chapter 3).

Don't take a caffeine-containing OTC drug on a daily basis, or you may wind up with a caffeine-withdrawal headache when you try to cut back on the pills. If you're having daily headaches, you need to see a doctor for an evaluation and help in setting up a migraine-fighting plan.

If OTCs don't help relieve your migraines, you may need to move up to the next rung on the pain-killing ladder — prescription migraine meds (see Chapter 5). Or you can try supplementing your OTC medications with alternative remedies.

Finding anti-inflammatories helpful

Nonsteroidal anti-inflammatory drugs (NSAIDs) are widely used for painful ailments. They come in both prescription and OTC form. The OTC forms include Advil and Motrin (ibuprofen), Aleve (naproxen sodium), and Bayer (aspirin). All of these OTC drugs can have side effects, including stomach irritation and bleeding, nausea, and vomiting.

Excedrin Migraine and Excedrin Extra Strength are staples for many people who have mild to moderate

Get me to the pills on time!

Camilla Pierce, a Houston homemaker and a migraine sufferer for 30 years, explains what works for her: "I've never
really known for sure what triggers my headaches exactly,
except for any intense physical activity like aerobics — and
that always does. I do know that any headache I had would
get very bad if left untreated. The only thing that has ever
worked for me is Excedrin. I've never had to use any kind of
prescription medications for my migraines."

migraines (both contain exactly the same meds). The
common side effect — stomach upset — may be an
acceptable tradeoff for pain relief.

If you're taking Extra-Strength Excedrin or Excedrin
Migraine, you're using a product that combines acetaminophen and aspirin with caffeine. With Aspirin-Free
Excedrin, you're taking acetaminophen and caffeine —
a combination that can provide pain relief for some
migraineurs.

Assuming that you're an adult who's not allergic to
NSAIDs (see Chapter 5 for more info on NSAIDs) or
any of the ingredients in Excedrin, and that you're not
pregnant, you may use it as your staple ammo for
most headaches. Then, on the rare occasion when the
going gets rough — and a headache turns into Bad Bad
Leroy Brown — you may need to turn to your tougher
backup: a prescription migraine troubleshooter.

Admiring Advil

When taken early in a migraine attack, Advil may
work well in relieving the pain of a mild migraine.

To stop an in-progress migraine, you can try Advil Migraine. Mild to moderate migraines often respond well to Advil Migraine, which is exactly the same as Advil Liqui-Gels. Both work faster than garden-variety Advil.

Sidestepping the Side Effects of Too Many OTC Drugs

Take too many OTC drugs, and you may be doomed to experience side effects such as nausea, vomiting, or the Eternal Headache, better known as a rebound headache (see Chapter 3). Furthermore, excessive OTC drug use can result in problems such as liver or kidney damage (depending on the medication).

So aim to be a savvy migraineur and safeguard yourself from overdosing. If you're using OTC remedies for a very bad migraine, find a way to keep track of the number of pills you're taking. If you're reaching for the pill bottle in the middle of the night — when you're half-asleep and reeling from pain — you may get confused and take more than you should (unless you have some kind of system for keeping track).

 One woman tells of setting out her just-in-case migraine pills at the start of her headaches so that she won't surpass the number that's safe to take in a 24-hour period. She uses a chart to help her remember when she took the first one, when it's okay to take another, and so on.

This advice may sound like simple connect-the-dots guidance, but the truth is, you can use all the help you can get when a pain stupor mutes your thinking processes. (You know this if you've been there.) And if a mate or friend isn't standing by to hand out pills, you'd better find your own way to deal with pain relievers in a safe manner.

As a general rule, you may be inviting disaster (a rebound headache; see Chapter 3) if you're taking the recommended dosage of a medication two to three days a week for several weeks.

Using Vitamin and Herbal Supplements

Vitamin supplements work well for many people who battle migraines. Because some headache experts now believe that a lack of sufficient magnesium is the culprit behind many migraines, the practice of smart-bombing migraines with supplements has become popular. Other vitamins can be used to bring balance to your body so that it's better able to combat migraines.

By the same token, some people are big fans of treating migraines with herbal remedies — a controversial option on which the jury is still out. You're probably not going to find many physicians who'll give herbal remedies a hearty thumbs-up. Not yet, anyway, because studies to illustrate that these supplements are safe and effective have been insufficient.

 If you're going to use vitamins and herbal supplements to help treat your migraines, you should be supervised by a doctor, and perhaps even a nutritionist. You need to have a health-care provider look at your entire health picture before you start taking a few fish-oil capsules here, a little magnesium there, and a few leaves of feverfew for a snack. Remember that all the parts of your headache game plan need to mesh neatly for the best overall pain-fighting effect. Remedies that aren't compatible can add some new symptoms to your troubles.

Taking your vitamins

Some migraine researchers believe that certain vitamin supplements can decrease your likelihood of developing headaches by balancing your system. Therefore, some migraineurs who are thrashing around for pain relief get very excited about the idea of taking vitamin supplements as a migraine remedy.

While vitamin advocates — and many doctors — support using vitamins to help get rid of migraines, many healthcare providers aren't convinced that nutritional supplements are beneficial for treating migraines. Also, the excessive use of vitamins sometimes can result in nasty side effects: Too much vitamin B6 can cause numbness in your hands and mouth; an overdose of magnesium supplements may affect your nervous system adversely, and magnesium intoxication can be fatal; and too much vitamin C can give you diarrhea.

 If you suspect that you have overdosed on vitamins, go to an emergency room or call your doctor. Some signs of vitamin overdose include:

- ✔ Cloudy urine
- ✔ Convulsions
- ✔ Dry lips and skin
- ✔ Frequent urination
- ✔ Irritability
- ✔ Itchy skin
- ✔ Lack of appetite
- ✔ Mood swings
- ✔ Muscle weakness

Seeking help when attempting to vitamin-bomb your migraines is a good idea. Headache specialists are good sources for advice on vitamin supplementation.

They're up-to-date on the latest studies, and they have experience monitoring patients who use supplements for migraine treatment.

Correcting dietary deficiencies may help your migraines as well as your overall health. Before you try any of the following supplements, get a doctor's advice on what supplements may be best for you (and what supplements will work with the medications you're already taking). Your physician takes into consideration your age, your past medical history, your current food regimen, and other factors that should go into the mix when deciding what supplements you need for deficiencies. But try to get most of your vitamins and minerals from food. Too many vitamins can be as dangerous as a deficiency of vitamins.

With each of the following supplements, the dose listed is the recommended daily dose for adults (*mg* is an abbreviation for *milligrams*). You can try using these supplements for your headaches, but if you experience negative side effects, back off on supplementation. You don't want to take vitamins that make you feel worse instead of better. (Incidentally, vitamin E is measured in IUs, or international units.)

✔ **Magnesium (400 mg):** Magnesium can be depleted by medications such as diuretics (called *water pills* because they reduce the amount of water in the body), alcohol consumption, and chronic medical problems such as diabetes. But if you eat spinach, nuts, bananas, bran, and whole-grain breads and cereals, you may get plenty of magnesium without taking a supplement. Symptoms of taking too much magnesium include diarrhea, drowsiness, and lethargy.

✔ **B2 (400 mg):** Studies have shown that 400 mg of vitamin B2 (riboflavin) can greatly reduce migraine frequency. One rare bothersome side effect of vitamin B2 is diarrhea.

✔ **Fish-oil concentrate pills (2,000 mg):** Fish-oil pills with 360 mg of the omega-3 fatty acid EPA (eicosapentaenoic acid) and 240 mg of the omega-3 fatty acid DHA (docosahexaenoic acid) are believed to reduce the intensity of an existing headache or help stave off headaches so that you don't have them as often.

✔ **Vitamin C (2,000 mg):** These supplements are usually sold in 1,000 and 1,500 mg pills, so you can take two of the 1,000 mg pills a day. Vitamin C is recommended for headache prevention.

✔ **Vitamin E (400 IU):** Vitamin E is good for circulation, and thus, helpful for some people who suffer from migraines.

✔ **Vitamin B6 (200 mg):** Some researchers think that vitamin B6 helps to ward off headaches. (Don't exceed the recommended dose.)

Tiptoeing through the herbal remedies

Herbal remedies are occasionally used as adjuncts to a central migraine-management plan. On the other hand, some people claim that certain herbs take care of their migraine pain entirely! (If someone swears by an herbal-only approach, check for a crystal ball and gypsy jewelry, because getting rid of a full-fledged migraine with nothing but herbal remedies ranks right up there with cleaning up an oil spill with tissues.)

If you're working on a migraine-management plan, and you're considering some form of herbal supplementation, be sure to consult with your healthcare provider.

 Don't imbibe gallons of the hottest gimmick coming down the pike until studies have proven its effectiveness. ***Remember:*** One person's anecdotal experience isn't enough to gamble your head on. Maybe the latest buzz around the water cooler is that drinking powdered ginger and water cures migraines! Hip-hip-hooray! But, on the other hand, some miracle migraine myth is spread among the populace just about every other day. Sure, the ginger cure may turn out to be true. Then again, it may be bogus.

Kava (or *kava-kava*) was all hot-cha-cha until there were reports that this herbal remedy made from the plant *Piper methysticum* may cause liver damage. However, you may still find kava for sale, and it may be labeled as a migraine remedy.

Herbal products aren't regulated for purity, so there can be variability in the amount of herb and impurities present.

If you just can't resist trendy remedies, check with your healthcare provider before taking them. If she gives you the go-ahead, you may want to sample some of the following herbal hotties:

- ✔ **Bayberry tea:** Some people use a cup of this drink as a headache deterrent when they feel a migraine coming on. If you still develop a headache after drinking it, try drinking another cup later in the day.

- ✔ **Chamomile tea:** This tea is a popular herbal treatment used to relieve migraine pain after a headache hits. It does double duty, because it also helps sooth rocky stomach woes. Drink one or two cups.

- ✔ **Feverfew:** Long used as dry leaves in tea to treat inflammation and swelling, and highly lauded as a migraine preventive, feverfew (the herb *Tanacetum parthenium*) reportedly helps many people. It's usually taken in capsule form. Follow the recommendations on the bottle for dosage. ***Remember:*** Feverfew doesn't work for everyone (of course, neither does anything else). When you stop taking it, you may get jittery and have trouble sleeping for a while.

- ✔ **Ginkgo:** Ginkgo biloba, believed to improve blood flow to the brain, may help relieve your headaches. ***Warning:*** Don't use ginkgo if you take *anticoagulants* (blood thinners), aspirin, lithium, or ergotamine with caffeine. Check with your doctor before using this or any other herbal remedy.

- ✔ **Lam Kam Sang Heklin:** This big ol' raw-herb hodgepodge is said to relieve migraines fast.

- ✔ **St. John's wort:** The herb St. John's wort *(Hypericum perforatum)* is sometimes used to reduce anxiety and depression and relieve headaches. ***Warning:*** Don't use St. John's wort if you're on birth control pills or prescription antidepressants, such as Paxil or Zoloft.

- ✔ **Valerian:** This herb is used for both anxiety relief and migraine pain relief. Keep doses low, because too much can make you hyperactive.

Using herbal remedies for migraine relief is very controversial. Most people think that for every person who gets help via an herbal remedy, there's another who tried the same thing and got no help whatsoever. (Could it just be a placebo effect?) The same thing can be said of acetaminophen or ibuprofen, although many studies have proven these medications to be effective. One person's surefire solution may be another person's live toad on the head.

Avoiding ephedrine

A headache is but one of many problems/symptoms that can result from taking supplements containing ephedrine. The U.S. Department of Health and Human Services warns consumers not to take dietary supplements containing ephedrine, because these products pose significant health risks, but they continue to be popular among health-club enthusiasts.

Marketed as weight-loss products and alternatives to illegal street drugs such as ecstasy, these supplements contain botanical (or so-called *natural*) sources of *ephedrine* — an amphetamine-like stimulant that can have dangerous effects on the heart and nervous system.

These products are marketed under many brand names, and labels promise or suggest that they can promote weight loss, produce euphoria, enhance sexual sensations, heighten energy, and so on. But these supplements may cause possible adverse effects that range from headache, dizziness, and heart palpitations to heart attack, stroke, seizures, psychosis, and death.

So stay away from products that contain ephedrine, which may be listed under one of many aliases: ma huang, Chinese ephedra, ma huang extract, ephedra, ephedra sinica, ephedra extract, ephedra herb powder, or epitonin.

Chapter 5

Taking Care of Pain with Prescription Drugs

. . . .

In This Chapter

▶ Finding relief for your headaches

▶ Knocking out a headache that's under way

▶ Preventing migraines altogether

▶ Using the superhero medicines

. . . .

*T*oday, doctors have a huge arsenal of headache
drugs that can prevent a migraine from getting
worse, stop head pain in its tracks, make recurrences
less likely, and even prevent a migraine from happening in the first place.

Because a migraineur's brain has overly sensitive cir-
cuits that overreact to stimuli that don't bother non-
migraine folks, calming down these mega-sensitive
nerve cells clearly is critical to pain relief. And that
became the job description of a migraine-combating
drug that gained U.S. approval in 1993 — sumatriptan.
Its success unleashed the drug class of triptans,
which have provided tremendous relief for many
migraineurs in the decade since.

But finding relief isn't always simple. Because migraines are very individualistic in pain level and frequency, and because people respond differently to different medications, you may have to try several prescription medicines to find the one that works well for you. You must hang in there until you find the right stuff, because the migraine-pain-relief options today are amazingly effective, and you have everything to gain from taking the time to zero in on your solution.

In this chapter, you find everything you ever wanted to know about various drugs for migraines. We familiarize you with their impact on headaches, their side effects, their likelihood to cause dependency, and their incompatibility with other meds and health conditions.

Looking for Relief in All the Right Places

Sometimes you get tired of hearing yourself repeat the same old refrain: "My head's killing me!" But it's hard to come up with creative phrases when you're writhing in pain (and perhaps nauseated, as well). The truth is, a migraine makes you desperate for answers, and your battle cry becomes the oft-repeated "Help me get rid of this head-splitting agony!"

So you turn to your doctor, and he introduces a whole field of dreamy medications designed to eliminate migraine pain. The only problem is, what works for one person may not necessarily work for you. So trial and error is the name of the migraine-med-sorting game.

The process starts when you huddle with your migraine-specialist doctor, and the two of you firm up a determination to devise a headache management plan — with both drug and nondrug remedies — that will help you ward off headaches before they take up residence in your skull, or fight them after they move in.

 No book can be a substitute for an in-person, one-on-one consultation with your personal physician, who knows all about your particular medical needs and conditions. Don't skip the consultation process!

Just to keep things interesting, the guide that many doctors use as a reference on drugs — a monthly booklet called *Monthly Prescribing Reference* — has a comment at the start of its migraine-drug coverage that says, essentially, that no one really knows for sure exactly how migraines work, so the way that many anti-migraine drugs work is only theoretical, and this is especially true when it comes to combination products.

 The information on migraine medications provided in this chapter is intended primarily for people who don't have special medical conditions in addition to their migraines, those who aren't 65 or older, and those who aren't children. If you fall into one of these groups, consult your physician for advice on appropriate ways to treat your migraines.

 Always check with a doctor before taking any drug! Don't take other people's headache remedies or improvise on your own medications. You must beware of any unusual migraine, because it may signal a more dangerous condition, such as brain hemorrhage, aneurysm, meningitis, or another life-threatening condition.

The name game

Understand that each drug has several names associated with it — not just to confuse you but to flesh out the persona and character of the particular drug. For example, a given medication has a chemical name that's rarely used but is reflective of its chemical composition, a descriptive class name, a generic (hard-to-pronounce) name that points to the drug family it came from, and a *trade name* — the registered name the manufacturer gives the drug — which is probably the one you're most familiar with. Some examples of trade names are Imitrex and Advil.

In the same way that you can call an automobile by a descriptive name (a steel, plastic, rubber, and chrome, human-steered, gasoline-powered vehicle), generic name (car), or trade name (BMW), you can also sort a medicine by its descriptive class name (serotonin receptor agonist), generic name (rizatriptan), and finally, its trade name (Maxalt). The true chemical name for a drug, which is usually a mile long, doesn't come up very often — fortunately.

Generalizing about drug types

In your investigation of drug therapies, you'll find that the arsenal of anti-migraine drugs features quite a variety, including the following:

- ✔ General pain-fighters
- ✔ Drugs that address migraine side effects
- ✔ Medicines made especially for migraines
- ✔ Medications that were originally created for other medical conditions but were found to help migraine pain, as well

The two overall categories for migraine-treating drugs are *abortives*, medicines that stop a headache that's already under way, and *prophylactics* (or *preventives*), drugs aimed at preventing a migraine from occurring. Prophylactics, by the way, aren't the first line of defense, simply because you don't want to take medication that you don't need — and a regimen of preventives requires a daily tablet in most cases.

Coming to terms with migraines

Certain words keep popping up in headache talks — so much so, that you really need to know migraine jargon to stay abreast of what's going on in the ever-changing treatment field.

To sort through all the pain relievers, though, you need to understand their "doctor names" — because physicians tend to toss these names about during headache-treatment talks. Take a look at the following list of common pain relievers:

- ✓ **Abortives (or abortive therapy):** Medications called abortives fight existing migraines. These pain relievers are also called acute medication, rescue meds, and relief drugs. They work to relieve pain after a headache arrives, whether it's just warming up or blasting your head like a rock concert. This category includes plenty of prescription drugs, as well as some first-line-of-defense OTCs (over-the-counter medications) such as Excedrin Migraine and Advil Migraine (see Chapter 4 for OTCs).

- ✓ **Antidepressants:** Certain antidepressants, which are frequently used to treat depression, have found a second role as migraine preventives. Some of these are Elavil and Pamelor.

- ✓ **Antiemetics:** These medications are used to control migraine-associated nausea and vomiting, but they can also help relieve migraine pain itself. Two antiemetics are Reglan and Phenergan.

✔ **Beta blockers:** These drugs, long used to treat high blood pressure, can also be used to prevent migraines. Examples are Inderal and Blocadren.

✔ **Calcium channel blockers:** Commonly used to treat people with high blood pressure, calcium channel blockers also work for preventing migraines, because they can establish a balance in your blood vessels and stave off oxygen deficit in the brain. Calan is an example.

✔ **Ergotamine:** The drugs called ergotamines, or ergot derivatives, can abort acute migraines because they constrict blood vessels, but more importantly, they block pain impulses from getting to the brain. In other words, this kind of drug causes a narrowing of the brain's arteries and diminishes pain. Examples of ergotamine-based medications are Cafergot, Ergostat, Migranal, DHE-45, and Sansert.

✔ **Monoamine oxidase inhibitors (MAOIs):** The MAOIs are antidepressants that are used for migraine prevention. Doctors don't usually choose MAOIs as the first line of defense, because they have the potential for interacting with so many different medications and foods, which can result in serious health consequences. If your headaches don't respond to other prophylactic treatments, your doctor may prescribe an MAOI. Examples of MAOIs are Nardil, Parnate, and Marplan.

✔ **Narcotic analgesics:** These medications contain an opioid (a drug that acts on the body just like opium and its derivatives), and therefore, they aren't available over the counter, but they can be used for severe headache pain. (These are different from regular analgesics described in Chapter 4.) Some opium-like compounds that are sometimes used for pain relief are butorphanol and oxycodone.

✔ **Nonsteroidal anti-inflammatory drugs (NSAIDs):** These are painkillers that people take for a number of medical conditions, including mild to moderate headaches. Used to address (and reduce) the inflammation that occurs during a headache, NSAIDs inhibit the production of *prostaglandins,* hormone-like substances that are known to cause pain. Some of the NSAIDs are Aleve, ibuprofen, and aspirin.

Remember: If you're pregnant or breastfeeding, ask your doctor before using NSAIDs. NSAIDs should not be used during the third trimester of pregnancy, because there's the possibility that the use of such drugs can affect the baby's heart. However, you can take acetaminophen during pregnancy.

✔ **Preventives or prophylactics:** You really have to love these meds, because they're the ones that can decrease the frequency of your headaches and perhaps even prevent them from showing up at all. Hooray! On the other hand, they don't work if an attack is already underway.

Preventives include prescription drugs and OTC drugs such as naproxen. You shouldn't start yourself on a daily regimen of preventive medication — treatment with preventives should be initiated by your doctor. Prophylactics include: beta blockers, antidepressants, anticonvulsants, and calcium antagonists.

✔ **Selective serotonin reuptake inhibitors (SSRIs):** The SSRIs are common antidepressants and antianxiety medications that can interact badly with some migraine medications, such as the triptans, and cause complications. Examples of SSRIs are Prozac (also available as the generic fluoxetine), Paxil, Zoloft, Celexa, Luvox, and Lexapro.

✔ **Triptans:** This term refers to medications that end with *-triptan,* such as the medicine sumatriptan. These prescription meds are often used as initial treatment for migraines.

Some of the nondrug terms your doctor may throw around include

✔ **5-HT:** This is serotonin, a chemical released in the brain that transmits signals between nerve cells and can affect the blood vessels in your head. Researchers believe that this substance plays a prominent role in migraine attacks because a narrowing of vessels (via serotonin) curbs head pain by blocking pain impulses from getting to the brain.

✔ **Caffeine:** Though harmful when overused (and the actual villain in caffeine withdrawal headaches), caffeine is only a trigger when someone gets too much, and then it can cause a headache. Otherwise, it constricts blood vessels and thus relieves pain.

✔ **Serotonin:** The fluctuations of this brain chemical are involved in migraine development.

✔ **Vasodilation:** When blood vessels increase in size.

✔ **Vasoconstriction:** When blood vessels decrease in size.

Fighting Back: Abortive Medications for Migraines Underway

You have a headache, you're hurting, and you want it to go away. This is where abortive drugs come in — they're the medications that can give an existing migraine a knockout punch. These pain relievers aren't intended for headache prevention.

Many abortive drugs can't be used for hemiplegic or basilar migraines. Hemiplegic migraines can cause temporary paralysis on one side of the body. If you have basilar migraines, you usually feel pain on the back of your head, and you may experience frightening symptoms, such as slurred speech, confusion, lack of coordination, nausea, double vision, vertigo, and even a loss of consciousness. This kind of headache can cause stroke, coma, and, sometimes, death. If you suspect that you have either of these headaches types, you should have your doctor evaluate you to rule out the possibility that your symptoms are indications of something worse. (See Chapter 3 for more on these headache types.)

The format used in the drug section is the brand name first, with the generic drug name in parentheses. In each category, we describe a sample drug (or drugs) in detail — one(s) commonly prescribed.

Follow your doctor's instructions on dosing. Don't take more (or less) medication than you're supposed to.

Nonsteroidal anti-inflammatory drugs (NSAIDs)

Often used for chronic pain, the NSAIDs are popular migraine remedies that come in both over-the-counter and prescription versions. These medications are actually used for both abortive and prophylactic treatment of migraines. Possible side effects include diarrhea, nausea, and stomach bleeding. Some examples are Advil, Motrin, Naprosyn, and aspirin.

Naprosyn (naproxen) is often used to relieve the pain of menstrual cramps and arthritis, as well as mild to moderate migraines. Aleve, Naprelan, and Anaprox also contain the same generic medication naproxen, but their dosing is different.

- ✔ **Mode of delivery:** Tablet.

- ✔ **Possible side effects:** Abdominal pain, peptic ulcers, gastrointestinal bleeding, heartburn, nausea, and sleepiness. Taking more than the recommended amount of Naprosyn can cause problems such as vomiting, drowsiness, and heartburn.

- ✔ **Don't use if:** You have had a bad reaction to aspirin, Naprosyn, or any other NSAID in the past. Don't take Naprosyn if you're pregnant or breastfeeding, you have liver or kidney disease, you have a history of ulcers, you take blood thinners, or you have clotting problems.

- ✔ **Doesn't react well with:** Aspirin, other NSAIDs, or blood thinners. Naprosyn also interacts with other medications, so be sure to check with your doctor.

Triptans

A group of drugs that totally transformed the treatment of migraines because of their amazing effectiveness, the triptans appear to affect a certain serotonin receptor in your brain that results in the constriction of blood vessels, but more importantly, they block pain impulses from getting to the brain. Possible side effects include dizziness, chest pain, and anxiety. Some examples are Amerge, Zomig, and Imitrex.

You shouldn't take triptans if you have cardiovascular disease (heart disease). And, unless your doctor evaluates you and suggests otherwise, you shouldn't take triptans if you have major risk factors for heart disease (such as diabetes, obesity, high cholesterol, high blood pressure, or a family history of heart disease), you smoke, you're pregnant or breastfeeding, you're postmenopausal, you're a man over 40 years old, or you're a woman older than 65.

In one study of 43 hospital employees, researchers at the Georgia Headache Treatment Center in Augusta, Georgia, compared patients using their regular therapy for 12 to 18 weeks followed by injections of sumatriptan as needed for migraine pain for six months. The number of migraine days patients got pain relief by using sumatriptan was 75 percent, whereas it was only 25 percent with their usual therapy. Lost workplace productivity (and non-workplace activity time) was 35 percent lower with sumatriptan therapy. This figure underscores the finding that treating migraines with sumatriptan improves pain relief, reduces lost workplace productivity and non-workplace activity time, and enhances quality of life.

The triptans can be used to relieve migraine headaches with or without aura, but they shouldn't be used for unusual types of migraine, such as basilar or hemiplegic migraine.

Amerge (naratriptan) works for a longer period of time than the other triptans, so it works well if you have trouble with recurrence of headaches. This medication is commonly used for migraines with or without aura, and it's often prescribed for menstrual migraines. You may take it any time after your symptoms begin.

- ✔ **Mode of delivery:** Tablet.
- ✔ **Possible side effects:** Nausea, dizziness, drowsiness, and fatigue. Although rare, serious cardiac problems may also result.

✔ **Don't use if:** You have basilar or hemiplegic
migraine (see headache types in Chapter 3),
heart disease, uncontrolled high blood pressure, a history of *TIA* (transient ischemic attack,
an episode of neurological dysfunction resem-
bling a stroke, but which resolves completely)
or stroke, liver or kidney problems, or if you've
taken other triptans or ergotamine-type drugs
within the previous 24 hours.

✔ **Doesn't react well with:** SSRIs, ergotamine-
type medicines, or triptans. Also, don't use in
addition to other triptans you've taken within
24 hours.

Frova (frovatriptan succinate), which became available in early 2002, is the newest triptan to receive FDA
approval for the treatment of migraines in adults.

✔ **Mode of delivery:** Tablet.

✔ **Possible side effects:** Fatigue, flushing, dizziness, dry mouth, chest and throat tightness,
and, rarely, serious cardiac problems.

✔ **Don't use if:** You have heart disease, a history of
stroke or TIA, uncontrolled high blood pressure,
or you have taken other triptans or ergotamine-
type drugs within the previous 24 hours. Don't
use for basilar or hemiplegic migraine.

If you have liver problems or risk factors for
heart disease, or if you're elderly, pregnant,
or breastfeeding, your doctor will consider
whether there's a better medication for you.

✔ **Doesn't react well with:** Other triptans, SSRIs,
methysergide, or ergotamines.

Known as an excellent first-line therapy, **Imitrex
(sumatriptan)** even works on tough headaches that
are hard to shake. It can be used for acute migraines
but not for basilar or hemiplegic migraines. You

should take Imitrex when symptoms first appear, but it may also be used any time during an attack. You often get relief within an hour or two.

- ✔ **Modes of delivery:** Tablet, nasal spray, injection.

- ✔ **Possible side effects:** Flushing, muscle weakness, dizziness, sore throat, drowsiness, neck pain, anxiety, agitation, headaches, itching, chest pain, sweating, and, rarely, seizures and serious cardiac problems.

  Too much Imitrex may cause such problems as sluggishness, tremors, or seizures.

- ✔ **Don't use if:** You have a history of heart disease, heart attack, angina, strokes, or TIAs, you have basilar or hemiplegic migraine, uncontrolled high blood pressure, or liver problems, or you've taken ergot-type drugs or any other triptans within the previous 24 hours or MAOIs within the last two weeks.

  If you're at high risk for heart disease (such as being obese or having diabetes, high blood pressure, or a family history of heart disease), you have kidney problems, or you're pregnant or breastfeeding, your doctor will consider whether there's a better medicine for you.

- ✔ **Doesn't interact well with:** MAOIs (such as Nardil), ergotamine-containing drugs (such as Cafergot), or the SSRI antidepressants (such as Prozac and Zoloft). Don't use Imitrex if you've taken any other triptan within 24 hours.

Maxalt (rizatriptan) is laudable for working soon after you take it, often within an hour or two. The orally disintegrating tablet form can be taken without water, because it melts on your tongue. Rizatriptan comes in both Maxalt-MLT (the melting tablet form) and Maxalt.

✔ **Mode of delivery:** Tablet (common tablet form and orally disintegrating tablet form).

✔ **Possible side effects:** Sleepiness, chest pressure, dizziness, nausea, fatigue, and, rarely, serious cardiac problems.

✔ **Don't use if:** You have heart disease, uncontrolled high blood pressure, basilar or hemiplegic migraine, or you've taken ergotamine-type drugs or other triptans within the previous 24 hours or MAOIs within the previous two weeks.

If you are pregnant or breastfeeding, have risk factors for heart disease (such as diabetes, obesity, or smoking), or have liver or kidney problems, your doctor will consider whether there's a better medication for you.

✔ **Doesn't interact well with:** SSRIs, MAOIs, methysergide, ergotamines, or other triptans. When taking propranolol, your dose of Maxalt should be lowered (consult your doctor).

Zomig (zolmitriptan) is a triptan that works fast and, for some people, helps relieve nausea.

✔ **Mode of delivery:** Tablet (common tablet form and orally disintegrating tablet form).

✔ **Possible side effects:** Dizziness, nausea, skin tingling, dry mouth, cold or warm sensation, drowsiness, weakness, trouble swallowing, chest or throat tightness, and, rarely, serious cardiac problems. Too much Zomig may make you feel sleepy.

✔ **Don't use if:** You have a history of heart disease, angina, or heart attack, uncontrolled high blood pressure, or you have taken ergot-type drugs or other triptans within the previous 24 hours or MAOIs within the previous two weeks. You should also avoid using Zomig if you have risk factors for heart disease (such as smoking, diabetes, or you're overweight), an irregular heartbeat, liver problems, or you're pregnant or breastfeeding. Don't take this medication for basilar or hemiplegic migraine.

✔ **Doesn't interact well with:** MAOIs, SSRIs, ergotamine-type drugs, or other triptans. Some drugs (Tylenol, birth control pills, Tagamet, and others) interact with Zomig, so check with your doctor before taking it.

Other triptans include Axert (almotriptan) and Relpax (eletriptan).

 Always check with your doctor for interactions with any medications you're taking.

Combination drugs

Named because they are, indeed, combinations of several drugs, combination medications often work well on migraines. Some examples of combination drugs are Fiorinal, Esgic, and Midrin.

 All combination drugs have the potential to make you feel sleepy. You shouldn't drink alcohol when taking these pills. And you must be careful not to exceed the recommended dosage (exceeding the dosage can lead to rebound headaches — see Chapter 3). The side effects of combo drugs may include the worsening of your headaches (if you use combination drugs too often) and possibly drug dependency.

Midrin (isometheptene mucate, dichloralphenazone, acetaminophen), which contains isometheptene, acetaminophen, and dichloralphenazone, serves to narrow dilated blood vessels that have been implicated in migraine pain. Midrin is commonly used for the treatment of mild to moderate migraines and menstrual migraines. You take it when you first notice symptoms.

- ✔ **Mode of delivery:** Capsule.

- ✔ **Possible side effects:** Dizziness, sleepiness, and rash.

- ✔ **Don't use if:** You have hypersensitivity to any of the components of Midrin (check the ingredients in the medication's literature), glaucoma, uncontrolled high blood pressure, severe kidney disease, liver disease, or heart disease, you've taken MAOIs within the previous two weeks, or you have had a stroke or heart attack. If you have high blood pressure, peripheral vascular disease, or are pregnant or breastfeeding, your doctor may want to consider other medication options.

- ✔ **Doesn't interact well with:** MAOIs and blood thinners. Also, be aware that Midrin's sedative effect can be increased if you take antihistamines, Valium, or another central nervous system depressant. Avoid taking Midrin with alcohol.

Ergotamine derivatives

Made from a fungus, these drugs constrict blood vessels in your brain. They sometimes cause vomiting, nausea, and muscle cramps. Some examples of ergotamine derivatives are Migranal, Cafergot, and DHE-45.

Cafergot (contains ergotamine tartrate and caffeine) can be used for migraines with or without aura. Take it when symptoms of a migraine first appear.

- ✔ **Modes of delivery:** Suppository, tablet.

- ✔ **Possible side effects:** Severe vomiting, elevated blood pressure, nausea, slow or fast heartbeat,

numbness, weakness, chest pain, and muscle
pain. Too much Cafergot may cause convulsions, headaches, leg pain, coldness in your
extremities, high or low blood pressure, vomiting, coma, or drug dependency. Ergot poisoning
can be a very serious matter.

✔ **Don't use if:** You have kidney or liver disease,
high blood pressure, heart disease, peripheral
vascular disease, allergy to drugs that contain
caffeine or ergotamine, or you're pregnant or
breastfeeding.

✔ **Doesn't interact well with:** Sudafed or any
drug that causes blood vessels to constrict,
nicotine or nicotine drugs that are used
for smoking cessation, beta-blocker drugs
(such as propranolol), or certain antibiotics
(consult your doctor).

Migranal (dihydroergotamine mesylate) is an
ergotamine-containing nasal spray that provides pain
relief by altering the amount of serotonin in your
brain and constricting blood vessels. It contains the
same active ingredient as the injectable form DHE-45.
Migranal is a good drug choice for combating migraines
that keep coming back. Don't use Migranal for hemiplegic or basilar migraines.

✔ **Mode of delivery:** Nasal spray.

✔ **Possible side effects:** Dizziness, drowsiness,
nausea, vomiting, nasal congestion, heart problems, and hot flushes. Too much Migranal may
cause ergot-poisoning symptoms such as
headaches, convulsions, muscle pain, numbness, or cold extremities.

✔ **Don't take if:** You have basilar or hemiplegic
migraine, heart disease (including angina),
uncontrolled high blood pressure, liver or
kidney disease, blood vessel problems (such
as Raynaud's phenomenon), you've taken

triptans or other ergot-type medications within the previous 24 hours or MAOIs within the previous two weeks, or if you're pregnant or breastfeeding.

✓ **Doesn't interact well with:** Other ergotamines, vasoconstrictors, triptans, MAOIs, and ery-thromycin. Migranal can also interact with multiple other medications, so let your doctor know all of the medicines you're taking. You should also let your doctor know if you have hypothyroidism, because Migranal may adversely affect this condition.

DHE-45 has the same active ingredient as Migranal. It's used for aborting severe headaches in a hurry. It's often given in injection form in emergency rooms to treat long-lasting migraines.

Corticosteroids

Usually the court of last resort for headaches that just won't go away, the corticosteroids mute your body's inflammation response. Possible side effects include anxiety and insomnia. (With short-term use of corti-costeroids, these side effects aren't usually a problem.) Prednisone is one example of a corticosteroid (see "Calling on Superhero Medications," later in this chapter).

Opioids (or narcotics)

These powerhouse painkillers are usually reserved for terrible migraine pain that won't go away after trying less potent pills. Side effects may include a sedated feeling, dizziness, vomiting, and sweating. The risk of rebound, dependency, and addiction exists.

Some examples of opioids are Percocet, Vicodin, and Demerol. (See "Calling on Superhero Medications," later in this chapter.)

Stopping Migraines Upfront: Prophylactics

During your info-gathering venture, you may become intrigued by the drugs called prophylactics, because they hold the enchanting lure of keeping migraines at bay entirely. Typically, if you tried avoiding triggers and using relaxation techniques and biofeedback, and you still can't control your migraines, your doctor may think that you can benefit from a regimen of preventive medications.

You're a good candidate for prophylactic therapy if you

- Have frequent migraine attacks (two or three a month), and they're so annoying that your quality of life is compromised.

- Have severe migraines that aren't relieved by forms of symptomatic treatment (treatment to relieve symptoms such as pain and nausea).

- Have menstrual migraine attacks that haven't responded to other methods of treatment. (A woman may be able to prevent migraine attacks by taking an NSAID a few days before starting her period, or during the first few days of menstruation.)

If your doctor thinks that preventive therapy is a good option for you, the goals are: less frequent headaches, less severe migraines, and improved quality of life.

But there are a number of reasons that you don't just jump willy-nilly into using preventives instead of trying to stop a migraine that has already begun. Check out the following downsides of prophylactics:

- ✔ **You need to be monitored.** Your prophylactic treatment has to be monitored by a physician, because each preventive medication has potentially dangerous side effects.

- ✔ **You're subject to side effects.** To reap the benefit (warding off headaches), you have to accept the possibility of living with side effects such as weight gain, hair loss, and so on. (See the descriptions of individual drugs in this section for specifics on side effects.)

- ✔ **You have to stick to a scheduled regimen.** This medicine won't relieve headache pain, so you have to take it every day to prevent a headache. Some people don't want to take drugs on a daily basis. Plus, prophylactic therapy just isn't necessary for those who only have occasional migraines.

Your doctor will usually start you on a low-dose migraine preventive and then gradually increase the dosage until it works well for you. Or he'll stop increasing the dosage if you find that the side effects become too annoying or you have reached the highest safe dosage. Don't give up on a drug and switch to another just because the low-dose version fails to help.

Some people find that prophylactics are very successful in preventing migraine attacks, while others find that they get less of an effect from the drug.

Prophylactics won't help a migraine already in progress.

Make sure that you follow a very specific doctor-prescribed schedule when taking prophylactics. Doing so will help prevent the spiral that starts a migraine. Along with taking the preventive properly, you should also eat a healthy diet, get enough rest, and exercise regularly to maximize the benefits of the drug.

The following sections cover some common groups of prophylactic migraine drugs.

Antidepressants

Antidepressants, which are actually meant for treating depression, have crossover appeal because they can also be used to treat migraines. Possible side effects include constipation, dry mouth, anxiety, elevated blood pressure, and weight gain. Some examples of antidepressants are Elavil and Pamelor.

Elavil (amitriptyline) is a tricylic antidepressant commonly used to treat depression, eating disorders, and chronic pain.

- ✔ **Modes of delivery:** Tablet, injection.

- ✔ **Possible side effects:** Sleepiness, dry mouth, constipation, weight gain, irregular heartbeat, impotence, nausea, and black tongue. Too much Elavil may cause convulsions, very low blood pressure, confusion, heart problems, or coma.

- ✔ **Don't take if:** You have hyperthyroidism, a history of seizures, liver problems, an enlarged prostate, glaucoma; you've had a heart attack recently; you've taken MAOIs within the previous two weeks; or you're pregnant or breastfeeding.

- ✔ **Doesn't interact well with:** Alcohol, barbiturates, carbamazepine, phenytoin, anticholineregics, guanethidine, and multiple other medications, so check with your doctor.

Pamelor (nortriptyline), a tricyclic antidepressant,
is most commonly used to treat depression and
chronic pain.

- ✔ **Modes of delivery:** Capsule, liquid.

- ✔ **Possible side effects:** Dry mouth, sedation,
  weight gain, irregular heartbeat, nausea, black
  tongue, breast enlargement, loss of appetite,
  and ringing in the ears.

- ✔ **Don't take if:** You have an enlarged prostate,
  hyperthyroidism, liver impairment, heart disease,
  glaucoma, you're pregnant or breastfeeding,
  or you've taken MAOIs within the previous
  two weeks.

- ✔ **Doesn't interact well with:** Mixing Pamelor with
  MAOIs can be fatal. Nortriptyline can affect your
  reaction to alcohol. Pamelor can also interact
  with multiple other medications, so be sure to
  stay in close contact with your doctor.

Antiseizure medications

Some medicines aimed at seizure prevention are also
good for migraine prevention. Possible side effects
include hair loss, nausea, and weight gain or weight
loss (depending on the medication). Some examples
of antiseizure medications are Depakote, Neurontin,
and Topamax.

Long used as an anticonvulsant, **Depakote (divalproex
sodium)** is also a successful migraine preventive.
Some doctors use Depakote first when dealing with a
migraineur who has seizures or certain psychiatric
problems. Depakote won't help a migraine that is
already under way.

- ✔ **Mode of delivery:** Tablet.

- ✔ **Possible side effects:** Weight gain, nausea,
  tremors, vomiting, hair loss, malaise, weakness,

facial edema, anorexia, drowsiness, and liver toxicity. Stop using Depakote and contact your doctor if bleeding, bruising, or a coagulation problem occurs.

✔ **Don't take if:** You have liver disease or you're pregnant or breastfeeding. Too much Depakote may cause a drugged feeling or coma.

✔ **Doesn't interact well with:** Blood thinners (warfarin), aspirin, oral contraceptives, barbiturates, erythromycin, rifampin, diazepam, and zidovudine. Depakote interacts with other seizure medications, as well as multiple other medications, so check with your doctor.

Your doctor will monitor the level of Depakote in your blood.

Ergot derivatives

Ergot derivatives are drugs that reduce inflammation and help blood vessels constrict, thus relieving headache pain. Ergot derivatives aren't popular for migraine treatment, because they can't be used if you have high blood pressure, heart disease, or certain vascular diseases.

 If you take ergotamine and experience numbness, tingling, muscle cramps, or coldness in your toes or fingers, call your doctor immediately.

A derivative of ergot, **Sansert (methysergide)** is a synthetic drug similar to ergotamine meds. It is used for migraine prevention, especially in people who experience disabling pain, but it's a last-resort migraine medication because it can have serious side effects.

✔ **Mode of delivery:** Tablet.

✔ **Possible side effects:** Nausea, vomiting, abdominal pain, weight gain, hair loss, insomnia, sleepiness, leg cramps, and, rarely, a serious condition that involves thickening of the tissue around the heart, lungs, or kidneys.

✔ **Don't take if:** You have heart or vascular disease, high blood pressure, thrombophlebitis, collagen vascular disease, or you're pregnant or breastfeeding.

✔ **Doesn't interact well with:** Imitrex and some other drugs (check with your doctor).

Don't suddenly stop taking this medication: You must be weaned over several weeks to avoid a withdrawal headache.

Beta blockers

The beta blockers, known for treating heart problems and high blood pressure, have proven to be crossover successes in the migraine-fighting arena. They help relieve migraines by relaxing blood vessels. Possible side effects include depression, fatigue, and dizziness. Some examples of beta blockers are Inderal, Blocadren, Corgard, Tenormin, and Lopressor.

Blocadren (timolol) is a beta blocker that has been approved by the FDA for the treatment of migraines.

✔ **Mode of delivery:** Tablet.

✔ **Possible side effects:** Fatigue, breathing problems, cold extremities, dizziness, slow heart rate, and chest pain.

✔ **Don't take if:** You have asthma or other lung problems, a slow heart rate, heart block (electrical disturbance in the heart), overt heart failure, heart or lung disease, low blood pressure, diabetes, hyperthyroidism, liver or kidney problems, lupus, or you're pregnant or breastfeeding.

✔ **Doesn't interact well with:** NSAIDs (the effectiveness of Blocadren will be reduced), ergot medications, calcium channel blockers, digitalis, quinidine, and other medications, so consult your doctor.

Inderal (propranolol), which is often used for treating angina and high blood pressure, is a popular migraine prophylactic. This drug requires careful monitoring by your physician.

✔ **Mode of delivery:** Tablet.

✔ **Possible side effects:** Fatigue, sleep disturbances, insomnia, breathing problems, low blood pressure, slow heart rate, dizziness, cold extremities, impotence, and depression. Too much Inderal may cause an irregular heartbeat or seizures.

✔ **Don't take if:** You have asthma, slow heartbeat, heart block, or overt heart failure.

Your doctor will consider whether there's a better medication for you if you're pregnant or breastfeeding, or if you have any of the following conditions: diabetes, hyperthyroidism, liver or kidney dysfunction, Wolff-Parkinson-White syndrome, lupus, or lung problems.

✔ **Doesn't interact well with:** Ergots, alcohol, other blood pressure medicines, antithyroid drugs, chlorpromazine, calcium channel blockers, theophylline, digitalis, haloperidol, cimetidine, plus many other medications, so check with your doctor.

Avoid stopping Inderal or Blocadren abruptly. Do not use either one longer than six weeks if it doesn't help prevent migraines.

Nonsteroidal anti-inflammatory drugs (NSAIDs)

Nonsteroidal anti-inflammatory drugs (NSAIDs) are used for abortive and prophylactic treatment of migraines. See the entry for Naprosyn under "Fighting Back: Abortive Medications for Migraines Underway," earlier in this chapter.

Monoamine oxidase inhibitors (MAO inhibitors or MAOIs)

Normally used for treating depression, the MAO inhibitors can also be used to treat migraines. They're occasionally prescribed for migraine prophylaxis. Possible side effects include constipation, dry mouth, weight gain, and insomnia. The downside of these medications is their many negative interactions with certain foods and drugs.

Nardil (phenelzine sulfate) is a MAOI used as a migraine preventive, but it's not used as much as other preventive medications, because it has so many possible interactions with drugs and foods. Typically, Nardil is used for the treatment of depression. In most cases, the drug's benefits are believed to be cancelled out by the risks (it can be fatal if you take it with certain other medications or certain foods!). Ask your doctor about side effects, medication interactions, and so on.

Calcium channel blockers

Calcium channel blockers, which were originally intended to treat high blood pressure and heart disorders, have been used to treat migraines with only mediocre success. They serve to interfere with calcium's ability to constrict blood vessels. Possible side effects include fluid retention, congestive heart failure, shortness of breath, and impotence. Some examples of calcium channel blockers are Isoptin, Verelan PM, and Calan.

Calan (verapamil) is a migraine-preventive calcium channel blocker. Verapamil is also marketed as Calan SR, Covera-HS, Verelan PM, and Isoptin. It is usually used to treat high blood pressure and angina. Some doctors consider Calan to be the best calcium channel blocker for preventing migraines.

- ✔ **Modes of delivery:** Tablet, capsule.

- ✔ **Possible side effects:** Dizziness, heart failure, constipation, nausea, low blood pressure, and flushing. Too much Calan may cause a drop in blood pressure and serious heart problems.

- ✔ **Don't take if:** You have low blood pressure, heart failure, sick sinus syndrome, heart block, irregular heartbeat or other heart or circulatory problems, muscular dystrophy, liver or kidney disease; you're pregnant or breastfeeding; or if you've had a bad reaction to a calcium channel blocker.

- ✔ **Doesn't interact well with:** Beta blockers, alcohol, ACE inhibitors, Tagamet, and multiple other medications, so check with your doctor.

Calling on Superhero Medications

Sometimes you have to bring out the big guns when you're fighting a migraine.

Superhero medications usually work well, but they have the downside of putting you out of commission, as they sedate you in addition to killing your pain. However, if you're suffering from a horrible headache, you may welcome sedation (or perhaps even a couple of smacks on the head) if you think that it will make you feel better.

Typically, if you're resorting to a superhero medication, you aren't too worried about whether you'll be articulate when doing a work presentation. Hampered by debilitating pain and vomiting attacks, you aren't even going to work. Work may not even be a distant consideration for the moment. The big issue of the day is simply ridding yourself of agony.

Heavy-duty pain-relief medications include opioid drugs, steroids, combination medicines that contain butalbital, and the injectable NSAID Toradol.

 If you're on one of the high-intensity migraine drugs, don't plan to operate heavy machinery, drive a car, or do anything else that requires hand-eye coordination and high alertness. You should also avoid making any serious decisions while taking these drugs. Plan on going to bed, letting the medication do its work, and falling asleep if you can. Hopefully, you'll wake up to find your migraine gone.

NSAIDs

Over-the-counter NSAIDs such as Motrin and Aleve may work for minor-league head pain, but they usually won't do the job for severe migraines. Prescription Naprosyn often works for mild to moderate migraines. But for emergency situations, the superhero NSAID Toradol is a strong medication for tough pain problems.

Toradol (ketorolac) works well for migraines that are moderate to severe. This drug is usually reserved for times when you fail to respond to other less potent meds. Toradol is used for migraines in the emergency room.

- ✔ **Modes of delivery:** Tablet, injection.

- ✔ **Possible side effects:** Nausea, dizziness, drowsiness, diarrhea, fluid retention, itching, and gastrointestinal bleeding and/or perforation.

- ✔ **Don't take if:** You have an allergy to aspirin or other NSAIDs, a history of peptic ulcers, a history of gastrointestinal bleeding or perforation, elevated potassium, low sodium, kidney failure, high risk of bleeding, or if you're breastfeeding. Also, don't take Toradol if you're taking aspirin, other NSAIDs, or probenecid. If you have liver or kidney problems or high blood pressure, or if you're elderly or pregnant, check with your doctor prior to taking Toradol.

- ✔ **Doesn't interact well with:** Toradol may affect the effectiveness of other drugs such as blood thinners, tranquilizers, certain antidepressants, diuretics, lithium, methotrexate, and ACE inhibitors (the blood pressure medications).

Opioids

Opioid drugs — narcotic pain relievers — can usually knock out headaches that are very resistant to treatment. When you're suffering with horrible head pain, that's very good news.

Opioid drugs (narcotic pain relievers) are used to knock out very resistant headaches, but they can make your nausea worse, and they'll definitely make you feel too drowsy to function normally. They also have the huge downside of carrying the risk of addiction.

Pain relievers that contain an opioid are often injected; they provide rapid pain relief. Narcotic analgesics used to relieve migraines include Demerol (meperidine), Stadol (butorphanol), and Tylenol with codeine (which comes in a pill form).

Demerol (meperidine hydrochloride) is used for severe migraine attacks or when you can't take other pain-relief medications.

- ✔ **Modes of delivery:** Injection, tablet, syrup.

- ✔ **Possible side effects:** Nausea, vomiting, sweating, drowsiness, constipation, and urine retention. Too much Demerol may lead to drug dependency, clammy skin, difficulty breathing, coma, seizures, and breathing problems.

- ✔ **Don't take if:** You have liver or kidney disease, thyroid problems, Addison's disease, irregular heartbeat, enlarged prostate, a history of seizures, a history of past or current drug abuse, or you're pregnant or breastfeeding.

- ✔ **Doesn't interact well with:** Tranquilizers, alcohol, antihistamines, certain antidepressants (the tricyclics), or MAOIs (when taken within two weeks of taking an MAOI).

Stadol NS (butorphanol) is sometimes administered in an emergency room or doctor's office when a bad migraine fails to respond to other medications. You get quick pain relief, and the effects last for several hours. But, you can get addicted to this painkiller, and building up a tolerance and having rebound headaches are two other possible downsides of Stadol.

- ✔ **Modes of delivery:** Nasal spray, injection, intravenous.

- ✔ **Possible side effects:** Drowsiness, sweating, nausea, and high or low blood pressure. Also, addiction, rebound, and tolerance.

✔ **Don't take if:** You have lung, liver, or kidney problems, heart disease, problems with drug abuse, or you're pregnant or breastfeeding.

✔ **Doesn't interact well with:** Alcohol and sumatriptan nasal spray.

Corticosteroids

If you have prolonged migraine attacks, corticosteroids may be a good solution. Prednisone, for example, is very effective.

Although **Deltasone (prednisone)** is effective for treating migraines, it isn't often used, because it tends to have more side effects the longer you take it.

✔ **Mode of delivery:** Tablet.

✔ **Possible side effects:** Mood swings, insomnia, increased susceptibility to infection, ulcers, and high blood pressure. Prolonged usage may lead to weight gain, osteoporosis, and multiple other problems.

✔ **Don't take if:** You have a fungal infection throughout your body, or with a live vaccination, such as an oral polio vaccine. Your doctor may want to consider other treatments for you if you have problems such as tuberculosis, kidney problems, diabetes, cirrhosis, history of peptic ulcers, or if you're pregnant or breastfeeding.

✔ **Doesn't interact well with:** Barbiturates, rifampin.

If you take this drug, your doctor will need to monitor your progress carefully. Discuss with your doctor the dosage, side effects, drug interactions, and precautions.

Decadron (dexamethasone) is used to stop migraine attacks that don't respond to any other treatment.

- ✔ **Modes of delivery:** Tablet, injection.

- ✔ **Possible side effects:** Mood swings, increased susceptibility to infection, ulcers, insomnia, and high blood pressure. Prolonged usage may lead to weight gain, osteoporosis, and multiple other problems.

- ✔ **Don't take if:** You have asthma, a recent heart attack, or a systemic fungal infection, or with a live vaccination. Your doctor may want to consider other treatments for you if you have problems such as tuberculosis, kidney problems, diabetes, cirrhosis, history of peptic ulcers, or if you're pregnant or breastfeeding.

- ✔ **Doesn't interact well with:** Barbiturates, rifampin, ephedrine, some diuretics.

Discuss with your doctor other aspects about this medication, such as dosage and other side effects.

Combination pain medications

Some of today's most effective and popular migraine drugs fall into the category called *combination pain medications*. These migraine drugs are so named because they contain acetaminophen or aspirin combined with another medication. The combo analgesics that contain a barbiturate or an opioid have habit-forming potential.

Fioricet contains acetaminophen, butalbital, and caffeine. These three components are also found together under the brand names Esgic, Anolor 300, and Esgic-Plus. (Esgic-Plus has a lower recommended dose.) **Fiorinal** differs from Fioricet only in that it contains aspirin rather than acetaminophen. The medications that are combined in Fiorinal are also found together under the trade name Isollyl. Fiorinal also comes in a preparation called Fiorinal with codeine, which has the same components of Fiorinal in addition to codeine phosphate. These drugs are meant for occasional use in the treatment of moderate to severe migraines.

- ✔ **Mode of delivery:** Tablet.

- ✔ **Possible side effects:** Drowsiness, gas, abdominal pain, dizziness, drugged feeling, nausea, and vomiting. Too much Fioricet or Fiorinal may cause headaches, confusion, sweatiness, liver damage, breathing difficulty, coma, or a physical or mental dependency.

- ✔ **Don't take if:** You suffer from depression, current or past drug abuse, an allergy to any of the components of the medication, porphyria, peptic ulcers, kidney or liver impairment, suicidal tendencies, you're pregnant or breastfeeding, or if you're elderly and/or debilitated. Also, you should not use Fiorinal if you have an allergy to NSAIDs, bleeding or clotting disorders, gastritis, thyroid problems, an enlarged prostate, or asthma. Fiorinal should not be used by teens who have chicken pox or flu.

- ✔ **Doesn't interact well with:** Fioricet doesn't interact well with alcohol, antihistamines, MAOIs, muscle relaxants, tranquilizers, and narcotics. Fiorinal doesn't interact well with alcohol, beta blockers, MAOIs, blood thinners, NSAIDs, oral contraceptives, narcotic pain relievers, tranquilizers, and other medications, so check with your doctor. You shouldn't drink alcohol or drive when you're taking these drugs.

Chapter 6

Living the Good Life Despite Migraines

So what's a migraineur supposed to do while she's waiting to get better? The enormity of the disability aspect of migraines is enough to take your breath away, not to mention mess with your mind. Plagued frequently with an aching head, you may feel dazed and confused, flummoxed and fragmented, conflicted and conflagrant. But, the truth is, you can live a normal life despite sometimes being hobbled by high-level pain.

You don't have to write off the fun part of life just because you suffer from migraines. Far from it. You only need to make a few adjustments to make sure that your nights of revelry aren't followed by days of blinding misery. You can discover how to deal effectively with the inevitable migraine blues. If you need to, figure out when it's best to become a migraine recluse — just go to bed and sleep off your pain. Figure out how to have fun despite the head-pain drawback.

Singing the Why-Me Migraine Blues

Migraines may make you feel sad and lethargic. Your appetite may be next-to-nothing, and you may have trouble sleeping. You may tell people close to you that you're depressed, because it's the only word you know that accurately describes the low mood of persistent head pain.

Don't be afraid to give yourself permission to hate migraines. After all, you'll only be in major denial if you try to pretend that you aren't irritated by having horrible headaches now and then. In fact, dealing with depression (or the blues) is an almost inevitable spin-off of being a migraineur. Anyone with any chronic illness (which migraines are) is at risk for depression. Researchers believe that having migraines may make you more susceptible to developing depression. And the flip side is true, too: Having depression makes you more likely to have migraines.

 Don't be surprised (or frightened) if your doctor prescribes Elavil — an antidepressant that is good at fighting depression and excellent for busting migraines. Antidepressants are not only used for fighting depression, they're also commonly used to treat people with migraines.

 If you're having symptoms of clinical depression, you need to see a doctor immediately. These symptoms include

✔ Despondent mood

✔ Lack of interest in normal activities

✔ Fatigue and low energy level

✔ Feelings of worthlessness or guilt

✔ Indecisiveness or inability to focus

✔ Insomnia or *hypersomnia* (sleep that lasts for long periods of time)

✔ Restlessness or a feeling of general slowness

✔ Significant weight loss or changes in appetite

✔ Suicidal plans or attempted suicide

✔ Thoughts of death

If you have five or more of these symptoms in a two-week period, to the extent that they interfere with your ability to function adequately and represent a change in your life that isn't the result of drug abuse, a medication, a medical condition, or a natural grieving process following the loss of a loved one, get evaluated immediately.

Switching focus to lose the blues

If you've had headaches for many years, you may be familiar with the migraine blues. But are you good at dealing with it?

A nurse we know found herself steeped in self-loathing every time she had to miss work with a migraine. She loved her job and hated the disability aspect of her headaches. "One day I decided I was going to fix my migraine grumpiness," she says with a laugh. "I knew I was driving my husband crazy, the way I grumbled all the time."

(continued)

(continued)

She sought the help of a psychotherapist, who asked her the hot-button question: "Do you really think you're worse off than most people?" "I felt so silly," recalled the nurse. "One of my friends has breast cancer, and another is going through the enormous stress of a lawsuit. Yet another is getting her third divorce." She admitted to the therapist that several of her friends had worse problems. "But knowing that really doesn't help," she said. "Getting outside yourself will help, though," the therapist said. "Look at some volunteer opportunities, and pick one. Then, make time for it. When you're feeling down about your migraine burden, go to the volunteer center and help some really unfortunate people."

She took her therapist's good advice and found that helping others did change her feelings about her own lot in life. "I still don't like having migraines, but I know how to shake the gloomy, blue feeling. Helping other people makes me focus less on myself. That makes all the difference in the world. I highly recommend trying this kind of thing."

Feeling Free to Get Pain-Free

Don't be afraid to take aggressive moves when battling migraine pain. Some people, despite their migraine misery, don't feel entitled to pull out all the stops when trying to nix head pain, mainly because of the stigma attached to drug use. Plus, they may fear that taking a strong pain reliever will make them feel even worse (the "dull brain" haze). Many people use heavy-duty medications to fight headaches. If these drugs work for you, don't let the stigma of the drug's name or strength level hold you back.

You may find it daunting to take antidepressants (the ones used to fight migraines) or seriously strong painkillers, because you feel like you're giving in to the fact that you need a formidable drug to knock out your headache. Remember, though, that lots of people have to take strong medications to keep medical conditions at bay or reduce symptoms of chronic illnesses. It's nothing to be ashamed of — just real life.

When deciding to take a heavy-duty drug, you should consider

- ✔ How well the drug works for you
- ✔ How tolerable its side effects are for you
- ✔ How liberating the effect of being migraine-free will be, thanks to the drug

Don't feel bad about occasionally using heavy-duty medication if that's what it takes to get rid of some of your headaches. After all, that's what these drugs are for. Just make sure that you follow your doctor's instructions for using the drug, and don't increase your dosage or your frequency of taking it.

 If you're lying in your bedroom writhing in headache pain, it's no time to be reticent about pain relievers.

 It's a good idea to have your doctor onboard when making all decisions concerning medications for headaches and any other treatments you may try, from herbal supplements to chiropractic treatments. You can feel safer and more secure with your physician monitoring your progress and answering your questions about side effects.

Deciding Whether to Go Out and About or Hunker Down at Home

One of the more difficult tasks for a migraine sufferer is figuring out how to deal with everyday life when suffering from a splitting headache. You ask yourself, "When can I manage a headache with medication and still get out of the house to do a few things? And when should I just forget about trying to do anything and fall into bed for sandman therapy?"

 Knowing when it's okay to leave the comforts of home is a key part of migraine management — it's not always an easy call. How can you tell if a course of action on a headache day is doable? The following list gives you some tips for gauging your prowess at taking care of business when dealing with a headache:

✔ **Assess your attitude for the day.** Don't take part in regular workplace or home activities unless you're pretty sure that you can stay on an even keel. (If you're going to be cranky with co-workers or your kids, you may be better off waiting until you shake the headache.)

✔ **Determine exactly why you're trying to get out and about.** If you're truly miserable with pain, but you feel like you have to strive for super-parent or super-worker status, stay home. You probably won't be able to accomplish anything, anyway; if you do, the effort will be at your health's expense.

✔ **Evaluate the effects of your medication on your ability to function.** Don't indulge in work or family errands or duties if your migraine brain haze can jeopardize your or someone else's safety: You should drive only if you have a clear head when you're taking your migraine pain medication. (If in doubt, check with your doctor to get her opinion on the safety of driving when you're taking a certain medication.)

Basically, your own personal experience will teach you what's workable with your pain-severity level. You may find, over time, that taking a pain reliever and then going about your usual routine can have a pain-relieving effect. Or you may have the opposite experience — discovering that your pain gets worse with any kind of activity.

Sleeping off a migraine

You may find that taking pain medication and sleeping off a migraine is the perfect remedy for your migraine pain.

If sleep works wonders for your head pain, don't hesitate to get some extra sleep. The fact that you sometimes snooze away migraine pain doesn't make you lazy, reclusive, or any of the other adjectives that an outsider may come up with. For you, a timeout or a day off may simply be the smart answer.

 Give yourself permission to do what you need to do. Take care of the business of getting rid of your headache. If freeing yourself from outside noise, light, and household confusion helps, it's definitely the right way to go. Snuggle up in a comfortable bed and let some good Z's bring you sweet release from your migraine.

Taking care of business with a monkey on your head

Thousands of migraineurs go to work with headaches. Thousands of parents continue carpools and grocery-store trips, even though they're suffering from headaches. Lots of people conduct board meetings, close deals, and give seminars while dealing with headaches.

 Here are some coping strategies for days when you have not-quite-incapacitating headaches:

✔ Take an over-the-counter medication that takes the edge off your pain.

✔ Keep the reassuring self-talk coming. ("I can run this errand and then go home and go to bed.")

✔ Set parameters for yourself. ("I won't try to work on that major presentation today; I can get through the simple stuff, but it would be foolish to tackle anything that requires extreme focus.")

Joining In the Social Whirl

From the time you were first diagnosed with migraines, you probably wondered exactly what it would mean for your social life. Do migraines automatically send you to the world of social nerdiness? Not necessarily. Actually, you can decide what you want to do and be, and then set your sights on finding a way to do those things. Thousands of migraineurs do it all the time.

Sure, sometimes you may have to cancel things. Feeling a bit of chagrin is natural, but remember that many people bail for other reasons, such as a virus, menstrual cramps, a family emergency, or food poisoning — the list goes on and on. So it's really not all that bad if you have to cancel sometimes.

Dating and mating

You set up a date, the big evening arrives, and those nasty migraine triggers team up and throw you a curve that escalates into massive head pain. You know that there's no choice but to take your migraine medication and go to bed — after calling your date to say, "I can't go anywhere tonight."

If the person you're canceling on happens to wind up as your significant other, she'll have to live with your migraines long-term, so why not see how her affection holds up from the get-go?

Everyone has problems that they cope with long-term. So try to have a sense of humor about having to cancel a date when you're suffering from a migraine. Tell your date that you feel bad — you have a migraine — but you'd like a rain check. Make it clear that the headache isn't an excuse — it's a reality.

You're going to be bummed, sure, but you can show an upbeat attitude: "When I have one of these, I usually feel better the next day, so I hope we can reschedule. It doesn't take long for me to get sick of being a shut-in!"

Partying down despite a party-pooper migraine

You *can* party. Yes, you can. "With monkeys biting my head?" you ask. How is it possible to love the nightlife when you're shuddering in a fit of pain? Is it really within the realm of reality?

Yes, you can sparkle, crack jokes, yuck it up, and do Britney Spears dance moves — *if your headache is on the way out*. Essentially, the only thing you have to do is decide whether you feel like you can party hearty and enjoy yourself. If not, don't push yourself, and don't go into denial; listen to your body talk.

If you know that alcohol is one of your headache triggers, avoid alcoholic beverages. Of course, you can expect a date (or mate or gal-pal) to urge you to "have just one," but stand your ground. You don't want to end up with a hammering head.

Get creative, and find a way to let your saucy party-self get out there when you do feel good. Make the most of your situation — don't be afraid to shake your booty!

Finding recreation you can enjoy

Thrash around for fun opportunities! If you're a migraineur whose system is easily nudged into Painsville, be sure to seize chances that allow you to make the most of your uptime.

 People with migraines usually develop a heightened appreciation for enjoying every single day because of their great awareness of the potential for many hours of downtime.

For every activity that you can't tolerate, there are literally thousands that you can tolerate. All you have to do is eliminate those few that you can't handle!

Intense aerobic activities are often troublesome for migraineurs, so you may not be able to soar as a snow skier, a triathlete, or a mountain climber. But you probably can be a dancer, a swimmer, a skater, a fast walker, a hiker, a yoga enthusiast, a knitter, or a gardener.

Here are some ways to weigh the headache potential for a recreational activity:

- ✓ **Consider the weather and setting:** Will the activity feature changes in altitude and weather, both of which are often migraine triggers? One study suggests that half of all migraines have weather changes as an ingredient in their inception.

✔ **Review the specific environment of the activity:** Will there be bright lights, loud noises, and strong fumes? A concert, for example, may merit your no-no list (unless you think ahead and make sure that you're not sitting by the speakers).

You can enjoy more recreational activities by working around things that may affect your migraines. For example, say that you're going to a birthday party in a Mexican restaurant, and avocados are on your migraine trigger list. You can simply take the alternative route of stuffing your soft corn tortillas with chicken, refried beans, and rice, and steer clear of guacamole, which is made with avocados.

Turning thumbs down on fireside chats

One migraine sufferer in an online support-group chat room said something that non-migraine folks may find unbelievable. "When I go on ski trips, I always get headaches sitting by the cabin's fireplace."

This statement only goes to illustrate the quirkiness of migraines. Something as seemingly innocent, benign, and delightful as a fireside evening carries at least three possible migraine triggers: hot chocolate, hot toddy, and the smell and smoke of the wood fire.

The message is this: Find out what can bother your system, and honor your body's preferences. If you're just dying to try something that you're unfamiliar with, be sure to have your migraine medication ready to go. Don't get caught unprepared!

Chapter 7

Ten (Or So) Ways Not to Treat a Migraine

....

In This Chapter

▶ Showing evidence of your migraine-savvy

▶ Making sure that you stay faithful to your management plan

▶ Sidestepping the trap of thinking that your migraine triggers are no longer triggers

....

*Y*ou know how it is with migraines — there are some things you can do and some things you can't. But one rule should be an out-and-out federal law: Don't repeat mistakes you made in the past. And that's what we mean by "ways *not* to treat a migraine."

To highlight the importance of relying on a valid headache plan (and not zigzagging madly into the land of improvisation), here are ten or so very important ways *not* to treat a migraine.

Go Off Your Program

Sure, you know that you get headaches from MSG. Or red wine. Or peanuts. But you still want to believe

that your triggers will lose their oomph someday.
This probably isn't going to happen. So it's far better
to stick to the migraine-management plan that you
devised — don't go veering off on side streets.

Methodical folks are unlikely to have trouble with
migraine pain after they get their management plans
worked out. But the wafflers of this world, the people
who experience a brand-new world almost every day,
are often too quick to abandon or forget the basics —
and oops, their headache does it again.

So try to be sensible and practical. You can't rewrite
your migraine-attack plan each time the weather
changes. Do what works, and stick to it.

If you pick up some new tips along the way, you can
incorporate them into your migraine-attack plan. But
don't go changing too much after you discover what
works for keeping your headaches in line. If your
migraine-relieving strategies have accomplished the
goals of reduced frequency and severity, why not
adhere to them?

Take Too Many Drugs

One day, you throw caution to the wind and take
someone else's drugs. Another day, you experiment
with several different medications during the several
hours that you're fighting a migraine.

Don't do it! Experimenting with drugs that aren't on
your migraine-management plan may result in nasty
drug interactions and perhaps even a horrible
migraine. You need to run your ideas past your
doctor and get an okay first.

Ignore Dosage Recommendations

You received some sound advice from a healthcare provider about how much of a certain pain-relief medication you should take — and how often. So, don't start improvising: "Oh, that helped a little bit, so I'll take twice as much an hour from now."

Don't do it! Knowing how much of your medication to take, and when to take that amount, is a critical part of getting good results. If you go jogging off the path of good medicine, you may end up with worse problems than a bad headache.

Believe Crazy Claims

"If you'll just put your head in the vise and let me drill a few holes, you'll never have migraines again." Off-the-wall treatments may sound intriguing, but be sure to run past your doctor anything that you want to add to your headache-treatment plan. Unless you have a medical background, you probably aren't qualified to weed through bogus product claims and pinpoint alternatives that are actually legitimate.

Sure, plenty of hucksters may want to sell you a crystal ball for predicting when a headache is coming, or a magic carpet that will zap migraine energy when you start feeling bad. But the truth is, you're going to find far more comfort in the kinds of treatments that have been validated for their helpfulness and safety in reducing the pain, nausea, and other symptoms of migraines. Let wacky witch doctors sell their bills of goods to someone else — you're not buying. It's best to keep your head intact — especially for all those days when you don't have a headache and your brain comes in handy.

Keep Taking a Drug That Doesn't Work

Don't keep taking a medication that isn't working or has never worked for you — it probably never *will* work. Nothing miraculous is going to happen just by virtue of your commitment to a certain drug. Instead, look for a replacement. Get with your doctor and try a different direction.

Try to Gut It Out and Go Out

When you're feeling very sick and incapacitated, you may try to keep a stiff upper lip, gut it out, and go someplace.

Of course, you don't want to miss anything, and that's a real motivator. But going places when you're way too sick is always a mistake. Chances are, you won't make it through the activity, and you'll be forced to cut the fun short and drive yourself home. Or you may wind up too sick to drive, and then you'll be in a real fix.

Stuff Yourself with Tons of Food

Migraineurs have been known to overeat, thinking that it may knock down their pain a few notches. They've tried everything else, for heaven's sake!

But food-stuffing won't do any good. The only reason your headache may seem to disappear right after you eat is probably just lucky timing — your headache is already on the wane. As a side note, packing on extra pounds probably isn't going to make you happy, either.

Try the Sun-and-Activity Remedy

Someone may try to convince you that you'll feel better if you just get out of bed and go to a festival or county fair. "A little sunshine, a beer or two, and a turkey leg, and you'll be as good as new."

Not so fast there. It isn't very likely that sun and full-tilt activity (or alcohol) will make you feel better if you're already in the throes of a bad migraine. In fact, these activities are likely to aggravate migraines.

On the other hand, if you have nothing more than the nagging edge of a headache, you may want to take some medication and go ahead with your plans.

Doctor-Hop

You don't like what you hear from one doctor, so you go to another, and another. Soon, you're making a hobby of it.

Seeing one doctor who focuses on your headaches and helps you find answers is a far better use of your time and money. When you find a medical advisor who understands you and can help you manage your migraines, stick with him. Pay attention to his suggestions until, together, you devise a headache-management plan that works for you.

Foster a Sick-Person Reputation

A gut feeling tells you that, despite what your doctor says, you really won't get well. You fear that you'll face debilitating migraines forever. Nothing is going to work for you.

One good way to make sure that you'll always have headaches is to get real comfy with the victim role and decide that all the coddling and TLC are pretty nice. If you take this approach, you'll only help give migraine sufferers a bad name.

Become an ER Junkie

For you, it's too much trouble to see a specialist and set up a migraine-management plan. Instead, you just head for the emergency room when you get a bad headache.

Bad plan. People who are frequent fliers in the ER have several big problems. The staff may begin to dismiss your complaints because you cry wolf too often. Furthermore, you may build up a tolerance to the medications you're given time after time. And, you may also become a drug-abuse suspect.

Take the time to see a headache specialist and find out the real scoop on what you should be doing — instead of just flying by the seat of your pants every time you have a migraine attack.

Diet, Health & Fitness Titles from For Dummies

For Dummies books help keep you healthy and fit. Whatever your health & fitness needs, turn to Dummies books first.

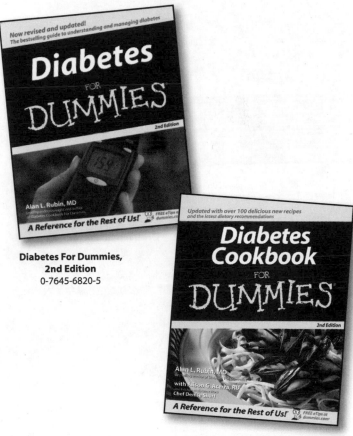

Diabetes For Dummies, 2nd Edition
0-7645-6820-5

Diabetes Cookbook For Dummies, 2nd Edition
0-7645-8450-2

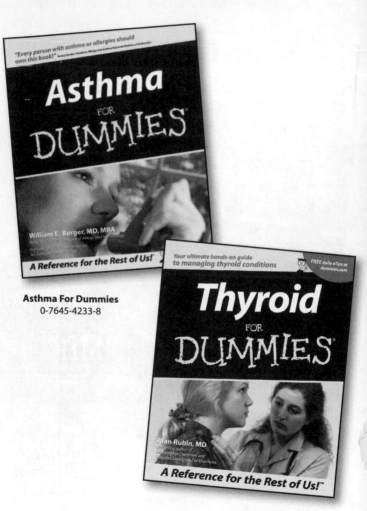

Asthma For Dummies
0-7645-4233-8

Thyroid For Dummies
0-7645-5385-2